Coping *with* Chronic Illness

H. Norman Wright
Lynn Ellis

HARVEST HOUSE PUBLISHERS

EUGENE, OREGON

Cover by Dugan Design Group, Bloomington, Minnesota

--- **ADVISORY** ---

Readers are advised to consult with their physician or other medical practitioner before implementing the suggestions that follow.

This book is not intended to take the place of sound medical advice or to treat specific maladies. Neither the authors nor the publisher assumes any liability for possible adverse consequences as a result of the information contained herein.

COPING WITH CHRONIC ILLNESS
Copyright © 2010 by H. Norman Wright and Lynn Ellis
Published by Harvest House Publishers
Eugene, Oregon 97402
www.harvesthousepublishers.com

Library of Congress Cataloging-in-Publication Data
Wright, H. Norman.
Coping with chronic illness / H. Norman Wright and Lynn Ellis.
p. cm.
Includes bibliographical references.
ISBN 978-0-7369-2706-2 (pbk.)
1. Chronic pain—Psychosomatic aspects. 2. Chronic pain—Alternative treatment. I. Ellis, Lynn. II. Title.
RB127.W75 2010
616'.0472—dc22
2009017211

Printed in the United States of America

10 11 12 13 14 15 16 17 18 / VP-SK / 10 9 8 7 6 5 4 3 2 1

Contents

Can You Relate?

I f you suffer from chronic illness...or know someone who does...you know how frustrating it can be. One day you feel relatively great...the next day you can hardly move or get out of bed because of the pain. One minute you're straightening up the house or garage and the next instant you're exhausted. Whether you're a man or a woman; whether your pain is physical, mental, or emotional; whether your up times outweigh your down times...or vice versa, *Coping with Chronic Illness* will encourage you and provide some ideas and suggestions you may not have considered. We've drawn on an extensive survey, a lot of conversations with chronic illness sufferers, Lynn's experiences with chronic pain, and my (Norm) knowledge based on my life and from helping people through my counseling practice. Although we don't know your exact situation, we understand how hard life can be when it comes to chronic pain and frustrations.

The following "life story" is a composite of many that people have shared with us while we were researching for this book. We're sure you'll be able to relate to many of the issues raised.

❧

I am female, age 49. Before becoming ill, I was an information systems manager in Northern California for a group of five hospitals. When I became extremely ill, I first thought it was a bad case of stomach flu, but it didn't go away. After months of testing, I was diagnosed with chronic fatigue and immune dysfunction syndrome (CFIDS) and fibromyalgia. I managed to continue to work for three more months, until it became impossible. I went on short-term disability in the month of May.

I lost my job and career in July. A three-year relationship with my significant other also ended in July because of my illness.

I lost my home two years later in September after my savings ran out.

I had to leave my community in November. I moved to Idaho to live with my parents because, by that time, I was destitute.

At the beginning of my illness, the medical community told me there was nothing wrong with me. It took more than a year of continuing to see doctors and having tests done to get any diagnosis at all. Once a diagnosis was made, I endured accusations from the long-term disability insurance company that this was a bogus diagnosis, that there were no such ailments. After all the medical testing, after racking up thousands of dollars in debt, after losing my job, my home, my community—I was told there was no officially recognized illness as CFIDS, and there was nothing wrong!

There is no cure for CFIDS or fibromyalgia. On one hand, I was relieved to have a diagnosis and have proof through specific blood tests that my immune system wasn't functioning. I had tests that showed inflammation throughout my body. But there wasn't much that could be done to help me. On the other hand, I was furious that after everything I'd been through, there were medical professionals who still insisted there was nothing wrong and CFIDS wasn't a "real" ailment.

On top of everything else, I was fighting with the Social Security disability people. My claim was denied. I appealed; it was denied, I appealed… and soon I was so exhausted and ill it was difficult to leave the house.

My greatest struggles thus far have been the tremendous losses. When this all began, and for the first two years after diagnosis, I nearly lost my mind. I had gone from the job of my dreams, which I'd worked 20 years to achieve, from buying my first home, from being respected in my field and my community, to losing everything. For the first couple of years, I seldom left my house. I was very isolated and suffered from situational depression. Side effects from the drugs I was prescribed made things worse. I felt total uncertainty over my future.

My parents, who had retired and settled in their home state, offered to take me in. They came and helped me pack, got me set up with a lawyer to wade through the Social Security mess, arranged for my home to be put on the market, and helped with all the things that needed to be done that I was too ill to take on.

I had been a workaholic my entire adult life. I truly believed my value as a human being was in my worth as an employee. I felt useless when I lost my career, especially when it became obvious I wasn't going to be able to work anymore. I remember my mom sitting me down, looking me squarely in the eye, and telling me I was a valuable human being just as I was. She didn't know why I was going through all this, but she assured me God had a plan that would be revealed. And until that time I needed to breathe in and breathe out over and over again if that was all I could do.

My experience with the medical community was pitiful for the most part. I had worked with doctors and surgeons for 20 years, many times directly, so it shouldn't have come as a surprise. When tests came back negative, I was told there was nothing wrong with me...that I was doing this to myself. My problems were all in my head, and I needed to "snap out of it." I had worked full-time since I was 16. I'd been working 14-hour days, six days a week for the last 2 years—and supposedly, all of a sudden, I'd decided for some unknown reason to convince my body to fall apart. This was their theory.

I finally found a physician who understood and was very helpful. His wife also had CFIDS, and they had gone through the same process I had. When I moved to my parents' home, we discovered a longtime family friend also had become suddenly very ill with similar symptoms to mine. She was able to get me into the Center for Special Immunology in Orange County, California. I fly down to California three or four times a year for treatment even now.

For the most part, I don't look ill. Fibromyalgia is a "soft tissue disease" affecting muscles, ligaments, and so forth. When it flares up it is debilitating. I depend on pain medication to make it through. In extreme flare-ups, it is difficult to walk; do basic tasks, such as showering and dressing; and stand long enough to prepare something to eat. But all days aren't like that. Some days I'm nearly "normal." People have a hard time understanding that I don't know from day-to-day what I will be able to do or how I will feel.

I've been living like this a long time now, and the people who couldn't or wouldn't understand went by the wayside long ago. The people who are in my life now do understand…or try to. They've been through this with me all these years. They know what kind of a day I'm having just by looking at me for a few seconds. They are very tuned in. I'm so very blessed with loving, compassionate family and friends.

To the people who don't know me well or don't understand, I try to explain. This illness has taught me to have much patience with others as well as myself. It has made me more empathetic and compassionate toward others.

My emotions? They run the gamut! Initially I experienced fear, sadness, confusion, anger, and grief. My diagnosing physician, the one whose wife also had CFIDS, told me before I left Northern California and moved to my parents' something profound that I listened to at the time but didn't really hear until much later. He knew I'd lost everything, and he told me this could be a real blessing—a rebirth, so to speak.

Yes, I had lost so much. I was really reduced to my basic self. I had nothing left to lose. Any step I took from that moment forward would be a new beginning. I would be with people who loved me unconditionally. I would be in a safe and secure environment. I would have an opportunity to truly begin again.

I fought this illness for the first several years. But now I've finally come to terms with the chronic nature of it. I am not this illness, this pain. I am a woman who has a chronic illness. I have learned each day is a blessing. My life is vastly different than the one I imagined for me, but all in all, it's a good one. It's also filled with challenges—but whose life isn't? My challenges are a chronic illness with chronic pain that I deal with on a daily basis. But now I can handle them and look for the beauty in the little things.

I am blessed with friends and family who are compassionate and loving and helpful. We lift each other up any way we can—with humor, with companionship, with keeping in touch, with sharing information. In the beginning, neighbors mowed my lawn, picked up my mail, brought meals, went grocery shopping, took me to doctor appointments and tests, kept in touch with my family, cared for my animals, and so on. I don't know how people in dire situations survive who don't have this kind of support. I don't know how I would have lived through these years without those nurturing souls.

In the beginning, many people couldn't understand the drastic changes in me and my life. It was very frightening to everyone—me included. My life was imploding, and I had no control. And when the debilitating pain went on and on and kept getting worse without a diagnosis or options for help, people felt helpless. The situation was very stressful. In fact, that's why my romantic relationship ended—the daily stress without relief was too much for him. He couldn't take it. I was also fortunate that I didn't have toxic people around me—negative people who would scoff and condemn me. The most hurtful people were the physicians who refused to take me or my health seriously so kept brushing me off.

I didn't have a church family in California, though I had a neighbor who was a minister and a dear friend. I don't have a church family here in Idaho either. I'm afraid I don't have much experience with the church. But how can people help me...or other people with chronic illness?

- Listen.

- Offer help and ask what is needed. It was very hard for me to ask for help. I'd always been the one to offer help and had never needed it myself. It was so difficult to ask for and accept help. But my friends persevered in supportive ways.

- Realize that a family member's illness affects the entire family.

- Be hopeful.

- Hold a hand or give a hug. Gentle human touch is very soothing and healing.

- Speak gently. I remember people who meant well would rage against my situation, saying it wasn't fair and it wasn't right. And that I wasn't being treated fairly by the medical establishment. All of this was negative and, even if it was true, wasn't helping.

- Recognize signs of depression.

- Recognize the power of prayer.

When my illness flares up, I still need help with the most basic things: bathing, meals, transportation. But for the most part, day-to-day, I just need reminders of how far I've come. When I feel overwhelmed by the pain, I need to be reminded it will pass. It always does.

I know I am where I'm supposed to be. For instance, if I hadn't come to live with my parents, I wouldn't have been in the position to help care for my grandmother, who is my light and my blessing every day. My family helped me get into a small house seven years ago. They spent six months taking this little "fixer-upper" and making it livable. My grandfather had passed away ten years ago, and my grandmother had been living by herself on their farm. When I moved here, so did she. She'll be 90 in July.

Our family helps us when we need it. Grandma has a church family she loves. (She's attended the same church since she was a little girl.) And we have the world's best neighbors. I have a group of 12 women—very diverse and in their 80s—I quilt with once a week. I've been with them for 12 years now. Many are widows. We are a family. We love and help each other. I take time every day to look—and to really see—the beauty around me. I have learned to listen, to be quiet, to find the comfort and the peace and the love that is around me. It has been a learning experience.

If I had not become ill, I imagine my life would have continued to revolve around my work. I would have continued to climb the corporate ladder to achieve "success," as I defined it back then.

I was given a chance at a different life. Not a life I would have dreamed for myself, but I've had lots of time to come to grips with my illness. Medication allows me to live with the pain. My health is as stable as it is likely to get. As my specialist said, "You're going to live forever; you're going to feel like crap, but you're going to live forever." Humor is critical; love is critical.

With a loving family and supportive friends and neighbors, I do have a positive outlook. I am where I'm supposed to be. A dear friend living with incurable cancer sent this to me two years ago. I keep it with me always.

> Turn out all thoughts of doubt and trouble. Never tolerate them
> for one second. Bar the windows and doors of your soul against

them as you would bar your home against a thief who would steal in to take your treasures.

What greater treasures can you have than Peace and Rest and Joy? And these are all stolen from you by doubt and fear and despair.

Face each day with Love and Laughter. Face the storm.

Joy, Peace, Love, My great gifts. Follow Me to find all three. I want you to feel the thrill of protection and safety. Any soul can feel this in a harbor, but real joy and victory come to those alone who sense these when they ride a storm.

Say, "all is well." Say it not as a vain repetition. Use it as you would use a healing balm for cut or wound, until the poison is drawn out; then, until the sore is healed, then, until the thrill of fresh life floods your being.

All is well.[1]

Be well and my best wishes to you.

1

A World *of* Pain *and* Frustration

There's an epidemic raging through our country. It's silent and raises no great alarm. Most people are unaware of it or they choose to ignore it. If you're reading this book, you're probably experiencing part of the epidemic. This illness takes over and regulates your life. Relatively invisible, it can't be seen like a broken limb or a visible deformity. This condition is one of the most glaring problems in health circles today, but it's largely discounted. In fact, you may feel ignored if you're suffering from it. Some people, including doctors and other medical personnel, believe if it isn't visible, "it doesn't exist." That's the prevailing mentality. Other than those struggling with the condition, few talk about the problem. What is this condition's name? Chronic illness.

Ninety million Americans had a chronic illness in 1987, and by 1998 it grew to 120 million. By 2030 it will probably be 171 million.[1] But the fact remains: Chronic illness (and the accompanying pain) is largely unrecognized.

"Chronic" is an interesting word, especially when it's linked to "condition" or "pain." A chronic condition has been defined as something that "is prolonged, doesn't resolve spontaneously, and is rarely cured completely." Can you identify with that? One doctor said that having a chronic illness is like having a career. You can do poorly or well at it. Doing well doesn't mean being cured; instead, it refers to your ability to cope and make needed adjustments. It's learning to live "in spite of." Some have lived well with chronic illness while others are crushed. Chronic illness means a life of uncertainty, including type of diagnosis (if any), treatment, duration, and what kind of future awaits you. Chronic illness is a life of certainty about having to face uncertainty, fears, and physical and mental anguish. Chronic illness means living with "invisible" symptoms that no one but you sees, feels, and are aware of.

As compared to diseases with clear-cut symptoms, chronic illness is often hard to describe accurately. You can't pin down what you're experiencing, which leaves you and others a bit puzzled. And it's difficult to measure some of the symptoms because of their complexity and the fact that some come and go without seeming to have a pattern. All of this lends itself to a diagnostic struggle. So does the fact that some symptoms could signify one illness or maybe another since they often overlap. Confusion exists in your mind as well as in the minds of medical professionals.

You may find it uncomfortable to talk about your symptoms with someone other than a doctor because of topic embarrassment: diarrhea, constipation, incontinence, cognitive impairment, depression.

Sometimes you may feel almost well, while other days you're incapacitated. This frustrates the people around you...and you. And you fear someday you'll remain incapacitated. Treatment may help...or may not...or may sometimes.

The diagnosis "it's all in your head" is a concern that comes and goes in your mind and in the minds of others as well. And in the minds of others some or all of the symptoms may seem nonexistent.[2]

How does chronic illness impact people? Listen to some who live with this illness:

- "It's been like taking some of your life away by taking pieces of it until there are so many things you used to be able to do that you can't do now."

- "It's just like when somebody dies. You grieve and you go through a cycle of disbelief, shock, anger, and so forth, but with this illness you end up like a hamster on a wheel where you just keep going around and around."

- "Why have any expectations? They just get crushed."

- "It's so different all the time. Today I'm fine and tomorrow it may be a different story. I could be knocked out. I have no predictability in my life."

- "It's not a typical depression. I'm dragged down by my pain and exhaustion."

- "I can't make big meals anymore. We have to limit the size of family gatherings."

- "I can't play racquetball anymore. I can't even clean one room."

- "I used to dislike going to work each day. I'd give anything to be able to work again."

- "I miss doing things for myself. I have to wait for others and I hate that."

- "I feel like a failure. I feel useless. I feel like a burden to my family."

- "My world has shrunk. I didn't choose this."

- "My struggle is keeping depression at bay. I'm on the edge of depression all the time and it doesn't take much to tip me into it. The illness goes in unpredictable cycles. When the illness is in a better cycle, the depression improves also. The other problem is trying to convince others that I really am sick when I look fine."

- "For years some of the doctors treated me like I had something mentally wrong with me. They prescribed addictive medications and then treated me like a drug addict if I called for a refill."

- "People don't understand and ask, 'Why do you go to bed so early?' If I don't go to bed at eight, I can't get up the next day. I can't do what everybody else can do, and when I try, I pay for it dearly. I have to learn to manage my life. I have to become my own doctor. And this is really hard."

- "When I woke up my head was killing me—my neck was messed up because of how I laid on my pillow. I have to be so careful—I just wanted to shoot myself because I laid on the wrong pillow and then I thought, *I can't believe this. I'm getting a migraine and I'm in this pain again.* I'm really disappointed. Then I think, *What do I tell others?* It's going to be disappointing for others and what do I tell them? I can just hear the conversation, 'How are you doing? How'd you sleep?' And I'll say my head is killing me, and I'm getting a migraine. It's such a letdown for me and it must be a letdown for others. So I'm struggling with what to do. Do I try and hide it or do I tell them because it's a disappointment for the other person? It's hard for me to deal with this, and it must be for them too. They're going to think, *Here we go again, another day—another headache.* It's just one of our struggles we deal with."

- "It's a feeling of being 'less than.' It's weakness."

- "Even saying, 'I'm doing the best I can with this disease' is a problem. Perhaps it would be better if this were a disease like cancer. But it's like these diseases don't count. Even in my mind they don't count as much. Some diseases are more acceptable than others. I have all these diseases that have been verified, but I still have a hard time with them being legitimate. It's like fibromyalgia is legitimate and yet it's not."

- "It's constantly working through these issues in my mind again and again, and it's a lifelong process. It's not like taking an antibiotic one time and it goes away."

Perhaps you identified with many of these experiences. Your story could be similar. Trying to make others understand your invisible illness is difficult. When others hear about it, they often say, "You look fine. It's hard to believe there's something wrong with you."

Your New Reality

What can you expect when you're struggling with chronic illness? Plan to be misunderstood by others. People don't understand what you're going through, especially because the illness can't be readily seen. They may judge, be indifferent, or show pity rather than support you.

Isolation may be another experience forced on you. Confinement isn't a pleasant experience. You may spend thousands of hours by yourself. This isolation soon turns into feelings that add to your misery. Rejection can lead to fear, loneliness, anger, and resentment. Many people are uncomfortable being around those who are sick and would rather be with those who are healthy. So you become isolated, which leads to feelings of abandonment and neglect.

You also may experience monotony. Because of your illness, reading or writing or watching TV may not be an option. Some find that any type of sound is stressful. The lack of activity and involvement can lead to guilt as well as a damaged self-esteem.

Have you ever felt dehumanized? When you're sick, you're soon seen as "sick" and referred to as "sick." If you're hospitalized you may feel dehumanized by the routine. When you feel you've lost control of your life, this feeling grows.[3] One woman describes her struggle this way:

> I was at the mercy of others. How easy it was to waver between guilt (for being such a burden), contempt (because help wasn't forthcoming), fear (that no one would be there if I needed help), anxiety (that if I asked for help, I would be rejected), anger (at my body that refused to cooperate), self-pity (that I couldn't function normally), panic (from things I didn't understand), dread (that I would get worse, not better), despair, hopelessness, worry, irritability, and frustration![4]

Imagine you're in a group at your church and several are aware that you have a chronic illness. One individual comes up to you with what seems to be a simple question, "What is a chronic illness?" That's an excellent question since most people don't have a clue. A chronic illness is "forever" (with a few exceptions) and is often painful. And what accompanies it is fatigue, depression, and a number of other symptoms, depending on the specific condition. Chronic illness necessitates constant involvement with the medical community, which is expensive. Your life is changed, often drastically. How? Alterations include your daily lifestyle, future goals, vocational choices, recreational activities, relationships with family and friends, and your role in your family.[5]

There are other words to describe chronic illness. Perhaps two of the most descriptive expressions we hear are "uncertainty" and "unpredictability."

And this is what is so frightening. We all function better with certainty and predictability. It seems no matter what you do or how hard you try, you're out of control. Your expectations, dreams, and desires for your body may go unfulfilled. And solutions are not forthcoming. When you have a chronic illness, you contend with a force that has more power than you. It's an illness with an agenda, which it knows and you don't. Chronic illness seems to have a mind and will of its own. It tends to scramble your thoughts as it ravages your body. You may settle into a routine, but it's not one of your choosing. And the routine isn't always routine. Actually there is little you can count on with your illness.

With chronic illness you no longer plan years in advance. It's hard to plan for the next day because you don't know how you'll feel. Your body, which you used to know so well and was a friend, has become a stranger and, at times, an enemy. The author of *Being Well When We're Ill* describes the situation so well:

> When chronic illness or disabilities invade our lives, we lose our dreams of well-being, of how we expected to feel each day, of what we anticipated doing in our later years, of what we intended to accomplish with our lives. Some of our dreams are replaced by better ones, but some of our losses leave us inconsolable.[6]

Chronic illness is strange. It doesn't fit the usual pattern of illnesses where you get sick with symptoms, see the doctor, get some medicine, and get better. There is no orderliness to chronic illness; it's chaos.

We've compiled a list that depicts what many people with chronic illness feel. You may want to circle the words that describe what you experience. Because of the changing nature of this illness, you may encounter many of them.

afraid	apathetic	chaotic
aggravated	apologetic	concerned
ambivalent	apprehensive	confused
angry	ashamed	damaged
anguished	belittled	defeated
anxious	burdened	degraded

dejected

dependent

depressed

deserted

despairing

devalued

devastated

disappointed

disconnected

discouraged

disheartened

dismayed

distracted

distraught

distressed

doubtful

embarrassed

excluded

exhausted

fatigued

fragmented

frantic

frightened

frustrated

furious

grieved

guilty

helpless

hopeless

horrified

humiliated

hurting

insecure

insignificant

irritable

isolated

lethargic

listless

lonely

lost

miserable

misunderstood

needy

nervous

overwhelmed

panicked

pessimistic

powerless

rejected

reluctant

resigned

sad

scared

self-conscious

sorrowful

stressed

tense

terrified

tormented

troubled

unnerved

unsettled

unsteady

unsure

upset

useless

violated

vulnerable

weak

weary

worn

worried

worthless

Chronic illness, with its accompanying pain, can result in private anguish. Others don't see your symptoms or pain. All they see are changes in you and may respond with anger, tension, or emotional withdrawal. They can't tap into what you're experiencing or how you feel. This may result in you feeling alone, abandoned, and trapped—with no way out and no help. It's similar to the reactions of those who experience grief over the death of a loved one for the first time. You may say, "I'm going crazy!"

When you live with chronic illness and its constant companion of pain, there's another resident as well: fatigue. You probably feel exhausted. Do you know what the word "exhaust" means? It comes from a Latin word meaning "to draw out of." Daily life is a struggle because you feel empty, all used up before you even get out of bed. Your resources are drained, and you feel 50 to 100 years older than you are.

So what do you do? You hang on to hope and concentrate on what you're able to do. You learn how to turn your life over to God's care and seek His comfort and strength.

For many with chronic illness, pain and fatigue become a constant. Admitting and accepting this doesn't equal resignation. In fact, it's more of a release! This is the first step of accepting the reality of the situation and discovering you are more than your illness.

Victory vs. Détente

Many images of illness and our responses draw on the language of combat: We *battle* illness and pain, *fight* infections, and *defend against* germs. Illness is an *enemy* to be *struggled with* and *defeated. Victory* over cancer is sought. Even fatal illnesses are to be constantly attacked in the hopes of medical advancements *(reinforcements).* The dying patient who wages a valiant battle to the death wins a resounding eulogy.

While chronic illness requires constant vigilance and may be reminiscent of war, ultimately there is no definitive battle to be won. There is no hill to take, no specific achievement to point to, such as remission or a cure. And a lifetime of being at war is extremely draining. Is a truce or détente the best we can hope for...or maybe a negotiated peace?

The way we speak about illness affects how we live with it. The war imagery obligates and even inspires us to resist. But chronic pain, which causes us to focus on surviving and coping, is often described using euphemisms such as "challenged" and "differently abled." This mutes the reality of the pain and suffering involved and can turn the natural sorrow, anger, and anxiety people experience into character defects, calling to mind defeat and resignation.

When you enter into the world of chronic illness you have so many decisions facing you of how to respond it's overwhelming. Each A or B choice contains risk and uncertainty. Which of these have you engaged in or considered?

A. You ignore symptoms, appear strong, and risk getting worse.
B. You overreact to every little twinge and pain.

A. You explore the possibility of a miracle cure, which could bring health and financial risks.
B. You choose to trust one doctor.

A. You keep your illness to yourself and carry the burden alone.
B. You talk openly to everyone, which could generate self-pity.

A. You demand that others treat you as normal, which doesn't allow them to share their concerns about you.
B. You let them cater to you, but worry about becoming dependent.

A. You push your body to override your illness so you "have a life" but you'll probably get worse.
B. You choose to be safe and overly cautious, which limits you.

A. You live with the fear of the worst happening.
B. You see each good day as a gift.

A. You choose to live with anger and resentment.
B. You focus on your blessings and perhaps risk a life of denial.[7]

When you have a chronic illness, your perception of yourself changes, and often not for the best. Some describe themselves as "deficient" or "defective" or they identify who they are by their illness: "I am fibromyalgia," "I am arthritis," "I am chronic fatigue," "I am lupus." This misidentity doesn't recognize their unique, God-given talents, skills, personalities, and characteristics. They need to separate their illness from who they really are.

A healthy response came from a woman who said, "I am not my fibromyalgia. I am a person not an illness. I am not just my hurting joints and muscles. I am more than this. I am more than my body. I am a choice person, a child of the King. I am loved just as I am."

How do you see yourself? How do you refer to yourself?

Remember, your illness may limit you, but it doesn't define you. Chronic pain may control some aspects of your life, but you are in charge of most areas...as well as your thoughts.[8]

Why Me?

Have you asked, "What happened to me? Why am I sick? Why do I have to suffer?" There are many reasons illness and disease occur. Some are physical—the immune system is too weak, too strong, or otherwise impaired. In a weakened state the strength of certain pathogens (bacteria, viruses, fungi, for example) is too much and overpowers the system. Or with an autoimmune disease, your system goes haywire and looks at certain good cells in your body as foreign invaders and says "they've got to go," so they're attacked by friendly fire. Why does this happen? No one really knows. It's a puzzle why these disorders exist, why some cells tell the immune system to attack, or why the system can't tell the difference between the good body cells and the bad invader cells.[9]

We're all aware that at some point in our lives we'll be sick. We hope that each experience will be temporary. If told that we have a disease, we hope it will be brief, pain free, and curable. If diagnosed with one that is permanent, we hope it is painless and not terminal. We hope it affects only the physical realm and not our mental capacities. We hope its symptoms are manageable and observable enough that they elicit support and sympathy from doctors, friends, and family.

But when chronic illness hits, the impact is total—body and mind. Often the mental stress is as painful as the physical. Most who live with a chronic illness will have additional struggles due to the reactions of people around them. Many will respond with help and support. And some are very knowledgeable. Some provide well-meaning but useless advice:

- "You really need to see this doctor. Everyone says he's the best, so don't waste your time with others."

- "You need to start treatment now before it's too late."

- "My stepsister has the same thing, and she's fine. It wasn't that painful for her."

- "Don't worry. It's in God's hands. Just remember Romans 8:28, 'In all things God works for the good of those who love him.'"

- "You have what? That disease will change you more than you realize."

- "This may sound strange, but this could turn out to be a real blessing in your life."

- "Have you ever thought that maybe God is trying to get your attention through this?"

- "You know, God only gives problems to those who can handle them."[10]

Knowing what comes next, in general at least, is a commodity we all want for security. With certainty, we can relax and move forward. Without it we're like a boat without an anchor, constantly drifting and running into rocks and underwater hazards. The statements just shared confirm our uncertainty, which leads to another struggle—doubt. What makes it worse is that it's self-doubt. You begin a continuous debate within your mind: "Am I really sick or not? Yes—no—I'm not sure. It feels like I am, but what if I'm not?"

Uncertainty takes an incredible amount of mental energy which, in turn, drains physical energy. And adding to your self-doubt are the responses of others, especially when you see suspicion and skepticism on their faces or sense them in their voices. The more you receive these negative responses, the more you tend to believe your doubts.

The best response is, "When in doubt, believe." You know yourself and your body. Document your symptoms by writing them down. Keep a journal. Believe they're true...because they are. The pain and symptoms are real. You're not dependent on others to validate what you are going through. They're not experts on you. Refuse to give others control over you. Yes, there are some aspects of your chronic illness you have no control over, but you do over your thought life.

Unfortunately, self-doubt won't exist by itself. Other negative varia-tions spiral, and sufferers end up not liking themselves. As one said:

> What's to like about myself in this condition? I question my
> condition and what I'm experiencing. If I can't be certain about
> that, how can I be sure about my own qualities and what I have
> to offer? Sometimes I find myself believing what I think others
> must think of me, and of course it's not positive.

Self-doubt creeps into your decisions about life, the future, and God.

> I look at others and they can rest in being certain about every-thing. My beliefs about God and who He is and what He does
> have crumbled. I wanted to get married, but that's not a given
> anymore. And how can I support myself? I can't even finish col-lege now, so the promise of the degrees and the profession I hoped
> for have vaporized. No wonder I don't like me or feel secure.

"Am I going crazy?" chronic illness sufferers ask constantly. You won-der, as do friends, family, and even doctors, "Is this real or is this all in my head?" With uncertainty, doubts about your sanity make inroads into your thought life. When a doctor hints or subtly suggests, "Perhaps it's more in your head than your body," and then asks if you've ever thought of seeing a counselor, self-doubt arises almost automatically.

When my (Norm) wife, Joyce, experienced her battle with fibrocitis (now called fibromyalgia) years ago, her doctor suggested she see a psy-chologist "just to make sure this is really a physical disease." She did... but it didn't make the illness go away. But just the suggestion fed her doubts.

Everyone has his or her own style of being sick. Does that sound strange? Perhaps, but we all "learned" how to be sick. Some of us want attention, and some want isolation. Some admit to being sick while oth-ers fight it and keep on going no matter what. When I was younger (in my thirties), I finally would admit that I had the flu and couldn't get out of bed. But I still wouldn't give up and give in. I even recorded a class lecture lying in bed and had Joyce take it out to the seminary and play it for my students. There are some people with chronic illnesses who are just as determined to not accept their conditions.

Think back to when you were a child. What did you learn about being sick? You learned how to behave when you were ill and what to expect from others. You developed beliefs about being sick. Some learned it's all right to express how they really felt while others learned to suffer in silence. Some learned how to use being sick to get what they wanted. Some received the attention they desperately wanted but never received when they were well. Some learned that in order to receive love, illness was the way. Others learned that the result of being sick was isolation and rejection. When you were a child, you also learned how to respond to pain. One woman said:

> I soon learned when I was sick as a child that I was seen as an inconvenience. I was tolerated because I was sick. Maybe I caused more work for them or maybe I disrupted their sched-ule. But I learned—keep my pain to myself. That was as bad as being sick. The problem is, what I learned then, I do now. It's so hard to let others know. I guess I started keeping all those experiences in my mind.

Your Experiences

1. Who were the caretakers in your life when you were sick as a child?

2. How did they respond to you positively?

3. What negative responses did you experience from anyone?

4. How are the messages or experiences from your past influencing your responses today?

5. How would you like to respond to people today regarding
your situation?

6. How would you like others to respond to you regarding your
chronic illness?

Affirmations

Read these affirmations aloud for encouragement. You might keep them
in a special place so you can refer to them when you're feeling down.

- I'm not alone with my chronic illness.
- I'm not the only one to think what I've been thinking or feel
  what I've been feeling.
- I can find new ways to respond to others to gain a greater
  amount of support and understanding.
- I can implement a new approach to accepting my illness and
  experiencing God's care and concern for me if I need to.

Prayer

*Merciful and healing Lord, for some reason which I do not under-
stand, the usual pattern of my daily life has been disrupted...*

Sit beside me now and help me to learn the purpose which this illness

*is to accomplish. Help me to see how much and how often I have
relied on my own strength, my own cleverness, my own ability.*

Forgive my pride that will not let me depend on You.

*In my illness help me to see that I am truly well when I remember
that I belong to You...Fill me with the life of the Spirit, that in
Christ I may be blessed and be a blessing to others.*

Hear my prayer in Jesus' name. Amen.[11]

∽◆∽

Recommended Reading

To learn more on chronic illness, we recommend these books. Some are
written from a Christian perspective, others are not.

Dawn, Marva. *Being Well When We're Ill.* Minneapolis: Augsburg Fortress, 2008.

Donaghue, Paul, Ph.D., and Mary Siegel, Ph.D. *Sick and Tired of Feeling
Sick and Tired: Living with Invisible Chronic Illness.* New York: W.W.
Norton & Co., 2000.

Edwards, Laurie. *Life Disrupted.* New York: Walker & Co., 2008.

Sverlach, Carol, M.A. *Just Fine: Unmasking Concealed Chronic Pain and
Illness.* Austin: Avid Reader Press, 2005.

2

The Search *for* *a* Diagnosis

Have you heard this diagnosis? "There is no clear answer. You have one of those conditions, those illnesses in which we just don't have anything definite. We're unable to make a diagnosis." Are you satisfied with this answer? Probably not. We're not sure anyone would be content with not knowing what's occurring within their bodies. That's one of the worst conditions we can ever experience. Our bodies are all we have on Earth. Our bodies are with us for better or worse, and if they're not working right, everything else, no matter how important, takes a backseat. We need answers—honest and accurate ones. And when they're not forthcoming, it's not just our bodies that are in a state of pain and tension, but our minds are as well.

Symptoms? What are they? Well, many can't be seen—they're invisible. Sometimes it's difficult to identify them because some of them are vague or intermittent or very general. It's hard to explain what you're experiencing when symptoms come and go and even you question whether they're real or not at times.

How does this affect diagnoses? Much of the time finding causes is not based on identifying a set of definite, measurable, observable symptoms, but by eliminating one possibility after another. This often entails multiple doctors and tests. As many have said, "I just want a name for my enemy." Frustration feeds fatigue, so that adds to the problem. Some people go for months and others for years in the wilderness of no diagnosis or "disease unknown."

Hidden symptoms are restrictive—as you are well aware. And that's one of the problems. Only you know of their existence. Others often don't "get it," and your former lifestyle now becomes a part of your history.

In time, others may pin a label on you—one that isn't to your liking. Many have said that as their illnesses go on, they become more defensive because of being misunderstood and labeled a hypochondriac. Symptoms can be silent thieves of your life and lifestyle. They steal your control, your desire to make plans, and your ability to carry them out. Commitments are broken more often than kept now, and nice days are becoming rare. And what about the other people in your life? Do they see you as sick or...

- complaining

- a hypochondriac

- lazy

- malingering

- overreacting

When you know how others perceive you, what do you usually do? Do you "fake it"? Try to appear normal? That's why many with chronic illnesses push themselves beyond their limits and then pay the price—symptoms made worse.

A Perception Problem

Living with an invisible illness is more difficult and stressful than living with one that is obvious. Some of your friends may disagree with this statement, but not you or others who live with chronic illnesses. Think about it. Notice the responses of others when they see someone who has an obvious illness or physical problem. You'll see concern, empathy, compassion, an offer to help or attempt to make something easier. They may or may not have pain with their disabilities, but others extend themselves regardless. Do you experience these positive reactions? Probably not—or at least not often—even though your suffering might be far worse than someone whose disability can be seen. Visible illnesses are taken seriously and at face value. You, on the other hand, may have to prove your illness and pain to others, which can be difficult. And why should you be forced to do this? It doesn't seem fair…because it isn't. Unfortunately, the reality is that for many, if a problem can't be seen, it doesn't exist.

Due to the vagueness, unpredictability, and variability of symptoms with some of the chronic illnesses, it can be extremely difficult to find answers for what is going wrong in your body. So the tests and exams continue. Sometimes you get a definite diagnosis, but other times you hear, "You *might* have…" Needless to say, this continual searching has an impact on your mental health. The constant unknowns cause you to question your senses and capabilities. The desire for certainty is ever present. Without knowing, you feel out of control because you don't know what to do to fix or cope with the problem. One of the worst feelings for any of us is the lack of control of some areas of our lives. It's even worse with chronic illness since there are multiple areas of little or no control—the illness, fatigue, the present, the future, and so forth.[1]

Don't deny what your symptoms are saying. Pretending to be well when you're not won't help. In fact, it usually makes it worse. Don't try to be an actress or actor. You won't get paid for it, and you'll end up paying the price—exhaustion and pain. Just think about it. If you look healthy, others think you're fine and expect you to perform as a healthy person. These unjustified perceptions put enormous pressure on you. You can try your best to fulfill their expectations, and then you experience a setback. Or you may make up excuses for your failure to meet their standards. There's a high cost for concealing illness. You may appear weak or inept. Trying to appear problem free and pain free is an arduous task.

Our advice? You can inform, but don't try to convince others of what you have or how bad it is. They'll believe you or not. And you can't control what they think or how they respond. You are who you are and have what you have. When you attempt to hide your situation from others, in a sense you're letting them control your life and who you are at this moment.

Proactive Solutions to Unrealistic Expectations

One of the suggestions I (Norm) have made from time to time to clients with chronic illnesses is to create 3 x 5 information cards. You describe in writing what you're experiencing and give them to those who ask you questions or when you meet someone with whom you're going to have ongoing contact. For example:

> My name is _____ and I have a chronic illness, which you can't see. It's not contagious. I didn't choose to have this illness. I wish I didn't have it, but I do and I'm learning to live with it. Please be patient.
>
> • Every day I experience...
> • The chronic illness limits me in...
> • When necessary, you can help me by...
>
> Thank you for your patience and understanding.

Symptoms create a battleground and Carol Sveilich, the author of *Just Fine,* puts it well:

> Most people with concealed illness or pain do not gracefully surrender. They valiantly do battle with their symptoms and yearn for their previous life. They fondly recall a time when a flight of stairs didn't seem akin to climbing Mount Everest. They long for a good night's sleep and a pain-free awakening. They remember easier times that didn't involve a perennial quest for a restroom. They miss earlier days when travel was not fraught with unpredictable symptoms.
>
> The battle to evade a new life with challenging obstacles usually persists until the body forces individuals to concede and make significant allowances for their symptoms.[2]

Living with chronic illness leads you to develop a new vocabulary. Some of your new phrases might be:

• "I would like to, but today I can't."
• "I used to be able to participate, but now I'm an observer."
• "This is who I am now."
• "I have a disease...but I'm not the disease."
• "Experiencing pain is *not* a sign of weakness."

It may also include saying no to your expectations and desires, and to others' expectations and desires as well.

Symptoms and the existence of chronic illness force you to develop a "new normal" for your life. This is necessary to create meaning in your life as well. Symptoms dictate that you let go of what you used to do and discover what you can do.

Your symptoms often generate responses that could easily defeat and immobilize you. One friend was told, "It's all in your mind." Instead of caving in to this suggestion and beginning to doubt and beating himself up mentally, he replied, "Well, yes and no. Some of my pain has migrated into my mind, but not as you're thinking. My mind isn't the source. It's more of a victim of what's happened to my body. So since my mind isn't the culprit, what other suggestions do you have for how we proceed now?"

Doctors Donoghue and Siegel, in their helpful book *Sick and Tired of Feeling Sick and Tired,* said: "There is much you can control and much you need to control in order to live as healthy and satisfying [life] as possible." You can control yourself in more mature ways. You can increase your self-discipline over your thoughts, focusing more on the present while avoiding the tyranny of "what ifs" about the future. You can control your ways of relating with others each day, growing more honest with your feelings, in understanding those around you, in deciding what to share regarding your needs and complaints. You can develop more positive, realistic attitudes and better handle negative, self-pitying ones. You can stop imprudent behaviors and learn those more conducive to your good health and well-being. You can eliminate your tendency to think you have no control.

> You need to have hope. While avoiding unrealistic hopes that you are cured during periods of remission or overly optimistic reactions to publicized reports of scientific breakthroughs, you can hope for an increased capacity to cope with your illness. You can hope to learn new ways of accomplishing tasks despite fatigue and pain. You can hope to accept your illness. You can hope to accept your illness more graciously. You can hope for patience and for growth in those qualities that make us more human, such as wisdom, courage, humility, generosity—qualities

that often have adversity as their sources and root. And you can hope for continued growth in peace, self-acceptance, self-appreciation and self-knowledge.[3]

There is hope. That's the theme of this book. We're not offering cures or radical changes in your illness or your lifestyle. But we are offering hope because we'll help you respond in new ways to your illness, access the "new mind" that Scripture calls upon us to have (Romans 12:2), and even see others responding and treating you with new understanding and acceptance.

The Good and Bad in the Medical Field

Your symptoms lead you to doctors and then diagnosis, which can be life-changing. Just imagine you're sitting across from your physician, who has devoted his or her life to the calling of medicine. Years of preparation and hundreds of thousands of dollars have been invested into this person you're basing part of your hopes on. Your doctor is trying to determine a diagnosis based on what you've said and what he or she has seen. You want answers. So does your doctor. You hope you'll hear conclusive words describing a nonserious, easy-to-treat, temporary ailment. It may happen...and then again it may not. Consider the possibilities:

- Your doctor may give you a quick diagnosis without running sufficient tests

- Your doctor may say, "I wish I knew, but right now I don't. We need to do further work."

- Your doctor may diagnose it quickly and accurately.

Who made the first diagnosis of your disease? You probably. In fact, you may have made a number of them in your mind. And you may have debated whether the first symptoms were even symptoms. But you knew something was wrong. At first the vagueness confused you. It's as though you're in a category of "well until proven sick." You may have debated with yourself whether you were sick or not. And then what happened if the symptoms pulled a disappearing act for weeks or months? Doubts dominated your thinking. You hoped for the best, but a sense of dread prevailed. And if tests are taken again and again with inconclusive results, confusion continues.[4]

The practice of medicine is not a perfect, infallible science. A wise doctor knows his or her limitations as well as those of medicine. A diagnosis can take time…much more time than you want to take. Test after test, many visits to the lab, and several trips to the imaging department may be part of your history as well as your future.

Become well acquainted with your doctor so you will have confidence in him or her. Some are skilled at diagnosis, while others are skilled at treatment. You want a doctor who is competent and insightful. Most physicians want to be known for that. It frustrates them too when no diagnostic answer is forthcoming.

The Effects of Diagnosis

Diagnosis. This word creates a multitude of feelings: dread, relief, grief, sadness, anger, confusion, devastation, joy, or a mixture of many of these. For some, it's the beginning of hope. For others, it's a confirmation that the life they once knew is truly over.

You may hear a diagnosis that you were afraid of hearing, and now you're in a state of semi-shock. You may not be ready or able to accept the news…similar to someone who has just received the news of the sudden death of a loved one. Only yours is the death of the life you knew and the unwelcome potential of an uncertain future.

What's it like to hear those life-changing words, "You have…"? Expressions of shock are usually the first response as your brain attempts to wrap itself around what you've heard. Diagnosis is a strange experience. It's supposed to answer questions, settle the unknown, and perhaps give some relief. But it's usually more of a disruption coupled with a sense of permanency. You may now have a name for your illness, but what baggage comes with this label? Does it bring certainty or more confusion and questions? Does it bring the desired relief or increased fear? Does it bring disbelief or validation? We've heard responses like:

- "I knew it. I just knew my life as I knew it was over. And there is no future."

- "I feel better knowing than not knowing, but it's still a shock."

- "I now have a name for this beast. I wish it could be tamed."

- "I'm still in shock and disbelief. It's like they were talking about someone else."

- "Actually my fear is better since I have a diagnosis...a name for it. My only fear is I hope they're right and it's not something worse."

- "I felt like someone dropped a load of bricks on me."

- "When I received my diagnosis I felt good. I felt relieved. I wasn't crazy. I was right all along, and all these others were wrong."

We all vary in our responses to the words of diagnosis, going from relief to grief. Some are cheerful while others are sad and morose. Some individuals feel fragmented, like a part of them was sick and a part wasn't. This is a way of detaching, a survival technique.

Your thoughts could be racing or just be stuck on one thing.

You might cry, pace, throw a fit, or sit in stunned silence staring at nothing.[5]

Once the diagnosis is in place, or even if it isn't, the phrase, "Let the games begin" rings true. Only these are mind games. Disbelief may be your initial reaction. "No! Not me!" "I don't believe it. This isn't happening to me." The emotional response to even seeking a diagnosis or receiving one can seem as destructive as the disease. It's not unusual to not want to know or to delay asking for the information. Unfortunately, some diseases left undiagnosed and untreated may quickly progress until treatment is no longer possible. So getting a diagnosis quickly is important. Your illness may be bad, but now you have some new companions—denial, fear, rage, anger, depression, anxiety, despair, guilt, shame, mood swings, and the feelings of helplessness and hopelessness. These responses, normal as they are, can be overwhelming and keep you from seeking the help you need and taking good care of yourself. You may become immobilized. For many, their lives are plagued with fear and their minds begin to concentrate on imagining the worst. Often your mind won't work the way it should. There's confusion, forgetfulness, lack of concentration, agitation, rigid thinking, and intrusive thoughts. Each emotion can feed the others and have a detrimental effect on your body's immune system. And the pain of feeling helpless often makes your symptoms seem even worse. Whatever initial responses of shock you have, they need to be faced and overcome. Don't let your disease *become the label of you as a person.*

Denial

Many people engage in denial—strong denial: so face the existence of denial. At some point in time you'll need to take action, but denial can help you not be overwhelmed by your illness. It buys you time to figure out what to do. But it's not helpful if denial becomes a permanent resident in your mind and heart.

Denial has many faces, some obvious and others not. One is simply refusing to believe the diagnosis no matter what. When you live there, you ignore the message your body is giving to you.

Denial also occurs when you over intellectualize, putting distance between you and your feelings (and your pain). You hide symptoms when you're around others. You're on stage performing a "wellness" act while your disease is at work tearing down your body. Denial has extremes— some choose to do nothing at all, whereas others become involved in every activity possible. They're constantly on the go and so busy they don't have to face the realities of their lives.[6]

Dr. Selma Breginty has identified seven levels of denial we use to handle bad news:

- *Level 1 is the Denial of Personal Relevance.* "Well, it might be true. I have a chronic illness, but it's not much. I can deal with it." Keep in mind the less threatened we are, the lower will be our level of denial.

- *Level 2 is the Denial of Urgency.* "This is a slow progressive illness. I have plenty of time. It will take years to develop."

- *Level 3 is the Denial of Vulnerability.* "I've met others with the same illness, and they're getting along fine. You can't even tell they are sick."

- *Level 4 is the Denial of Feelings.* "So what if it interferes with some of my activities. I can find something else to do."

- *Level 5 is Denial of the Source of Feelings* (and is tied into the previous denial). "I know I've been tired and cranky, but believe me, it's not related to my illness at all."

- *Level 6 is the Denial of Threatening Information.* "The doctors were telling me how it could affect me. That's just speculation at this point. I don't believe it."

- *Level 7 is the Denial of All Information.* "If you want to believe that, then I'm shocked. There's so much misinformation about fibromyalgia, you can't trust it. Some don't even believe it's real."[7]

Perhaps the following is similar to your story.

> Denial became a part of my life. I believed if I ignored my symptoms and pretended this had never happened, perhaps the pain and symptoms and fatigue would disappear. I even seemed to hide my symptoms from myself as well as others. But it wasn't to be then or now. I became the great pretender, but that's all it was—pretending. What I wanted was based on a false hope.

Adjusting with Action

Chronic illness disrupts your life in every way imaginable. You feel like you aged twenty years almost overnight. You may also identify with the words of this woman:

> My old self, the one whose skin I had always felt comfortable in, had departed. A new self was taking over my old territory, and I had to uncover a way to make peace with her. The challenge came in trying to force my old way of functioning into this new body and weakened state. This new self, the one that was struggling with fatigue, chronic pain, malfunctioning organs, and sleep deprivation, seemed to be affecting and infecting my career and personal relationships.[8]

Anger will probably visit you again and again. Diagnosis can do that. You may become angry at:

- how others are responding to you and not meeting your expectations
- people who tend to do too much or attempt to control you
- not being able to be diagnosed
- having your diagnosis changed again
- the doctors for lack of answers
- the economic costs your illness has created
- yourself for not responding the way you think you should
- those who are healthy and going on with their lives
- your body and its limitations
- feeling better one day and then worse the next
- not enough caring people
- others who can't read your mind
- God[9]

A diagnosis is like a good news–bad news scenario. It gives you some answers (both good and bad), but it can create a multitude of new questions and concerns. Not all of your questions will have answers, and this could continue throughout your lifetime.

In the long run it's best to have a diagnosis rather than a set of vague complaints. You need this for your peace of mind, your family's peace, insurance demands, employees or employers, and disability compensation. But remember: You are not your diagnosis. You are more than a disease. Don't refer to yourself by your diagnosis. Neither do you want to let your friends and relatives refer to you or define you as a disease (such as introducing you: This is so-and-so, and she has fibromyalgia).

A diagnosis will be of assistance in letting others know what's wrong, but don't let it limit you in the way you choose to live your life or stop your doctor from looking further into your condition. Too many people have shared with us the experience of going to a doctor with an ailment and having it attributed to their fibromyalgia or lupus or chronic fatigue syndrome without looking further into other possibilities. When you experience a new symptom, consider the possibility that it could be part of your disease...but it could be something else as well.[10]

What can you do? The first step is getting a second opinion or even a third. Be sure to see a specialist. After diagnosis, treat your disease for what it is—a life-altering loss. View it as a loss. Realize that you may be the only one who sees it as a loss, which means support for your grief may be minimal. Write about your feelings. Identify your worst fears. Pour out your anger and frustration. And learn as much as you can about the disease on your own and with supportive friends. Talk with others who have the same or similar diseases and benefit from their journeys. Find people who are grieving and *moving forward,* and avoid those stuck in their illnesses.

In the best of circumstances and in an ideal world, each of us would like to receive from doctors a "DD"—a dream diagnosis. Imagine how you would respond if you received your diagnosis this way:

1. Clear, conclusive diagnostic tests show that you have a serious health problem; however, there is plenty of hope. We will explore every avenue of cure and control until we find what works for you.

2. You can help by educating yourself about your health problem. Here is a list of books and Websites that will give you useful information.

3. There are many choices—many options for you to consider in your journey of rejuvenation. Here are a few for you to look at, and I hope you will find others that we can consider together.

4. I will offer opinions and give you the benefit of my experience and knowledge; however, the final decisions about your treatment are up to you.

5. I will spend all of the time you need right now to answer your immediate questions. Then there is a former patient waiting in my office whom I'd like you to meet. Three years ago she was given the same diagnosis I just gave you. Today her health

problem is under control. I think you can learn from her experience.

6. Listen to your body; it will be the best guide for both of us in this journey.[11]

There are doctors who are this thorough. Hopefully you will find one.

Remodeling Your Life

There are two responses to a diagnosis. You can allow the label to dictate how you live your life or you can use it as a launching pad to create a new life. Instead of being immobilized, you can use it to build a different life. With any major loss in life you don't return to how you were. A "new normal" is built. Norman Cousins was diagnosed with ankylosing spondylitis and given just a few weeks to live. Twenty years later he was still alive. He said, "Accept the diagnosis, but do not accept the verdict that comes with it."[12]

There are also two ways to live after your diagnosis: by fear or by hope. One we succumb to as it creeps into our lives, while the other is a deliberate choice that takes a daily commitment.

When you receive your diagnosis remember that *you are not the disease.* It doesn't define who you are. You have been afflicted with a life-altering disease, and the choice is yours as to what you do with it and where you go from here.[13]

> The diagnosis that you have been given is not a death sentence. It is an invitation to rebuild your life in a new and meaningful way. For people living with a debilitating disease, the message of hope can be as powerful as the cure.[14]

Jack Hayford offers you some words of hope:

> When you come to the end of any day that's been a hard day, it's usually as difficult to conclude as it has been to live. The end of the day can be the start of a long night of reliving the day's struggle and of missing the restorative powers of sleep through the restlessness of a night as bad as the day. So in seeking to lay

hold of this last principle, letting Jesus discipline us to navigate beyond hopelessness to hope becomes all the more important.

This is especially true when you know the day you're ending might not be much different from tomorrow!

Hopeless "days" can be weeks long, and the constituted agenda may not be rapid in its passing. Some things never go away fast enough, and the soul—the heart, mind and emotions—can become preoccupied to the point that they wheel over and over with the same cycle of thoughts, the same pinching of pain, the same specter of fear or the same bewildering doubts—all of it attended by the relentless question, "When will all of this go away?"

To find hope for a hopeless day—indeed, to conclude that bad day—is to place it into the hands of God and leave it there.[15]

Recommended Reading

We encourage you to continue reading on this subject and recommend the following books. Some are written from a Christian perspective while others are not.

Dawn, Marva. *Being Well When We're Ill*. Minneapolis: Augsburg Fortress, 2008.

Gruman, Jessie, Ph.D., *AfterShock: What to Do When the Doctor Gives You—or Someone You Love—a Devastating Diagnosis*. New York: Walker & Co., 2007.

3

The People
in Your Life

You aren't alone in your illness. You may feel that way at times…and maybe with good reason. But there are others who will help you if you enlist their support and derive the most from their presence. Let's consider your doctor first. In a survey, we asked respondents to describe their experiences with healthcare providers.

> "I have had six doctors after becoming ill—it was slow onset—mainly through my early thirties. I've had Western doctors, treating just my symptoms, and holistic doctors. I found it very irritating that some did not listen to me when I told them something was wrong. I was even told once I may be psychosomatic. I finally found a doctor who is both holistic and skilled in Western medicine. She also listens to me."

> "Wow! That's a hard one. For years some of them treated me like I had something mentally wrong with me. They prescribed addictive medications and then treated me like a drug addict if I called for a refill. Right now I am blessed with a wonderful Christian doctor who has never made me feel like that. He is very understanding."

> "Well…not always good. Some thought fibromyalgia just didn't exist. I would just agree…and say…sounds fine to me. I'd rather it not exist so I'll go with that. But here are my symptoms…and thousands share them…So, what do YOU think it is? I've heard

some really stupid things from some really educated men. I just crossed those doctors off my list."

"Doctors…the older I get the younger they get—and they don't understand polio, which is a disease of the past. Nor do they understand post-polio syndrome. Over the years, I've learned I must "educate" myself and physicians. I saw one neurologist who told me that post-polio syndrome was a cop-out for laziness and that I needed to push myself harder, which is the exact opposite of medline searches and PPS literature. I am constantly networking and reading about PPS. Doctors are humans and do not have all the answers. I'm thankful that I've had mostly good doctors that are willing to study and learn more about my disease."

"Generally I've been blessed by the doctors. Most try to be helpful and seem informed. I've learned I must be a bit assertive. Especially about medications they want me to 'try.'"

"Sometimes my doctors were matter-of-fact and clinical, but usually knowledgeable about the issues I'm dealing with. There are not enough MS specialists out there though. A neurologist can help me understand aspects of why my nerves are affected a certain way, but he or she doesn't understand the incontinence. Similarly, the urologist understands the incontinence, but not how the usual treatments work (or don't work!) with a person who has MS."

You and Your Doctor(s)

Let's consider how you can benefit the most from your experience. The first step is considering your level of understanding of your condition. Do you need to learn more? Do you wonder why you need to know so much about your illness? One reason is that it's not just your doctor who will treat your illness—but both of you together and for some time. When two individuals "marry," it's necessary that both are knowledgeable about marriage for it to work and to last. To receive the most benefit from the medical profession, you need to increase your knowledge of your illness. You may *want* others to make your decisions for you, but this is your life. You have to live with the diagnosis and results of your illness and treatments. You need to be aware as much as possible of your illness so you can understand treatment options. You'll also cooperate more with the recommendations if you understand the reasons for them.

Educate yourself about the various treatments so you can obtain the best care possible. This means making sure you've received the proper prescriptions and your records are correct. Always double-check prescriptions, number of pills, printouts, and so forth to make sure they're accurate.[1]

You have a choice of being either a "blunter" or a "monitor." Blunters have little interest in learning more about their illnesses and their prognoses. They try to keep their anxiety away by not facing the facts. Monitors are uneasy with the unknown so they search out as much information as possible.[2] Do you identify with either of these?

In preparation for your medical consultation, formulate a comprehensive list of questions regarding your condition. Never be afraid or hesitant to ask questions! Be sure you take them with you in written form. Here are some suggestions:

- What is the technical name of my illness?

- What does this mean? In what way does this disease or condition affect my body? What are the typical symptoms?

- How would you evaluate the state my illness is in?

- What causes this condition? Can there be more than one cause?

- What will cause this illness to progress or get worse? Is there any cure for this that you're aware of?

- What is the typical time course for its progression?

- Does my medical history or my family's say anything about my illness?

- What tests and procedures are commonly used to determine the course of treatment?

- What are the various treatments available for this condition?

- What are the effects of each treatment? Do they cure this

condition? How often do I have treatments? Do they slow
down its progression? How much?

- What complications and side effects are common and uncommon with each treatment?[3]

- Are there psychological changes that might occur? If so, what are they?

- If medication is prescribed, will they make me hyperactive, depressed, or sexually dysfunctional?

- What relational changes might I expect to occur?

- What effect could this condition have on my family, my ability to work, my service at church and in my community?

- From your experience, what will be my greatest adjustments?

The one individual who needs to know the most about your illness
and condition is you. Be aware that when you go to the doctor, some
may or may not have the specialized training to diagnose and treat your
illness. Educate yourself so you can engage him or her in a *partnership*
about your condition. You need discernment to sift through what you
will hear. An abundance of patience will also be necessary because an
accurate diagnosis and treatment can be painfully slow to arrive at. You
will be the one who will make the final decisions about your healthcare
and physicians. But be prepared to hear conflicting advice.[4]

Good doctor–patient relationships are an indispensible part of a successful diagnostic journey, and the relationship, eventual diagnosis, and
treatment options depend on compatibility and communication. Like
a first date with someone, the first appointment with a physician tells
much: Does the doctor look you in the eye when you tell your history?
Does he or she ask probing follow-up questions that show understanding and care? Subtle cues can reveal a lot.

There is a direct, critical difference between hearing and listening, and
you can usually tell early on what a new physician, specialist, or consultant is doing. When a doctor hears, he may be looking for confirmation
of what he has already decided. When he listens, he integrates your perspective on your body with his clinical one.[5]

What do you really know about your doctor? If you're like most of us, probably very little. What is his (or her) specialty? How long in practice? What medical school did he graduate from? What additional training or internships did he complete? How many others has he treated with this condition? These are just a few basic questions to consider.

Medical research and knowledge are advancing at a rapid rate. Doctors need to work hard to keep up-to-date on the latest advances, and many do. It's all right to ask what the latest research and findings are on your condition. It may be helpful to ask what books, resources, associative or support groups your doctor recommends to help you deal with your illness.

You also need a doctor with a good reputation in people skills as well as competency. Look for one who encourages questions rather than being threatened by them.[6] There are many knowledgeable doctors with great expertise available, but you need to do your part to find the best one for you. Here are some questions to ask yourself and the doctor:

- Does this doctor specialize in the treatment of my illness?

- Does he (or she) already have patients with my illness? How many has he treated?

- What kinds of alliances does the physician have with other healthcare professionals or hospitals? How connected is he?

- Are there other people in his practice who can assist in my care?

- What kind of health insurance does the doctor accept?

- What kind of communication skills does this doctor have? Do I feel comfortable in his presence?

- Would it upset the doctor if I sought a second or third opinion?

- What does the doctor think of alternative therapies?

- Does he listen to what I say and answer my questions in words I understand? Does he call back when I need assistance or information?

- How convenient is the office to my home and workplace?[7]

Doing Your Part

Help your doctor help you! He or she needs you to provide detailed information. *Always, always* do two things: 1) Go to your appointment with your information records, questions, and concerns in writing, and 2) take a pen and writing pad with you. If possible, have an advocate go with you (which we recommend) to write down what is said. The notes your friend takes are vital. Consider taking a tape recorder to use, but you will need your doctor's permission.

What can you do to help your doctor assist you? Prior to your visit, make a list of all of your symptoms—even those you wonder about. Prioritize them in order of importance to you or which are the most bothersome. List your major concerns and what you would like to say when asked, "How are you?" Don't hesitate to describe even those symptoms you think may be unimportant.

Here are some suggested questions and comments:

- How long have I been feeling this way? (Be as specific as possible.)
- As I see them, these are my symptoms…
- This is what has changed from my usual state of health.
- This is what I have gained or lost in weight.
- This is what I do that causes pain or discomfort…
- My symptoms are worse in the…
- When I run a fever, it usually gets up to ___ and lasts ___.
- My sleep has/hasn't been affected.
- The stress in my life is ___ and comes from ___ and ___.
- These symptoms have changed my daily life by…[8]

When you're with your doctor and he (or she) uses words you don't understand, don't hesitate to ask him to explain. Your task is to become educated about your illness, and that will include some medical terminology. Since it's in your body, learn everything you can about it and then some.

A prepared patient is a wise one. In fact, it's best to be over-prepared.

The following questions are for you to consider asking to increase your knowledge and understanding of your illness. When it comes to your diagnosis, ask and then ask again if necessary:

- "How is a diagnosis usually made?"
- "How certain is this diagnosis? Could it be anything else?"
- "Is this a common illness?"
- "Is it possible to get copies of the test reports, such as labs or MRI?"

When you discuss treatment be sure to ask:

- "What are the treatment options?"
- "Is it best to proceed quickly or wait a while?"
- "What are the side effects of the treatment or the medication?"
- "If this doesn't work, what are my options?"
- "With this treatment (or lack of) what is the prognosis?"

To gain the most from your appointments with your doctors, don't go alone. Take a trusted family member or friend with you. Let the person know in advance exactly what you would like him (or her) to do or not do. If you want the information to remain confidential, be sure you get his assurance that he won't discuss your situation or the content of the consultations with anyone else, including sharing the information as a prayer request. There may be an occasion when this person takes a dominant role or just a helping role, but since you're the patient, let him know your boundaries.

We've had some ask why this is necessary. Sometimes what you hear is a shock, and you can't fully absorb what is said. Even if it isn't, retaining all the details is difficult. An advocate or partner can bring up what you've forgotten or failed to put on your list, as well as take notes for you. Your ability to listen and understand may not be the best at this point. You may be hesitant to question or disagree with your doctor, but not so your advocate. Whoever you bring with you may be more objective and bring a balance into your perspective since you may tend to be optimistic or pessimistic.[9]

What about a second medical opinion? This is one of the best suggestions, and there's a good reason for it. Misdiagnosis is a fairly common occurrence. Research has shown that obtaining a second opinion results in a new diagnosis in as many as 30 percent of all cases. However, only 20 percent of those who seek medical care each year bother to get a second opinion.

Diseases commonly misdiagnosed are those often associated with vague symptoms that mimic other diseases. A few of these are chronic fatigue syndrome, which doesn't have any specific laboratory diagnostic test; depression that can cause a variety of physical and emotional symptoms; fibromyalgia, which like many other illnesses can cause a wide range of symptoms; thyroid disorders, such as hypothyroidism, which can cause vague symptoms such as fatigue and weakness. Ask your doctor for a referral. Other sources of assistance are available from medical societies or organizations that focus on specific illnesses such as the Lupus Foundation and the MS Society. "Doctor Finder," a referral association offered by the American Medical Association at www.Ama-assn.org, is another resource.[10]

To Share or Not?

Not only is chronic illness a source of pressure, but its presence creates yet another source of stress—who to tell about this, as well as what *they* should tell and what *they* need to tell. The question "How are you?" which used to be so simple and easy to answer, has now become something major. What you say in response to the question puts pressure on you as well as the person asking. Your answer may negatively impact your relationship. You have your own feelings to manage, but you also have to be aware and deal with the feelings of others about what you share.

Some people say it's just not worth sharing the details. Because they avoid talking about it, their energy goes into concealing their illnesses. If you do this, the misuse of energy puts even more stress on you because you have to be on guard constantly. Living a life of secrecy and protection isn't easy. The reasons for concealing vary:

- "I don't want to bear the label and stigma of being 'sick.'"

- "I don't want to answer intrusive questions."

- "I've been hurt too many times by insensitive comments."

- "I've already lost several friends over this, so why lose any more?"

- "I want to retain who I am...my original identity."

- "I don't want to be known as a whiner or a complainer."

- "I can't let those at work know because it would affect my job and any hope of advancement."

- "I don't want to be seen as 'less than' and have others talk about me behind my back."

Fear of losing the acceptance of others is a major cause for concern. No one likes to be rejected, and this can happen even within the Christian community. This should be the last place to expect rejection, but it occurs. Clichés, platitudes, spiritual advice, misquoting of scripture, and even judgments have wounded many. So people use the pat phrase of "I'm fine" to conceal what they're feeling and to silence others.[11]

If you decide to tell how you really are feeling, "who" and "how" needs to be considered. Your sharing may be highly selective, with a large amount of editing occurring. Some use "protective sharing," which means you expend effort managing who, what, when, and how you share. Others are totally open with everything about the illness and how they're handling it.

Disclosure is risky. It's not just deciding who to tell or what to share, but considering what responses you might hear. It may be doubt, rejection, disbelief, avoidance, support, or compassion. Mary described her feelings: "I felt as though I was coming out of the 'closet' with some socially unacceptable disease." Disclosing means you are willing to experience a change in a person's perception and response to you.

If your illness is one that will never become visible to others, you might struggle with "Why tell? If they can't see it, they'll never know, will they?" We've had some share with us if they had to be sick, they would rather have an illness that could be seen so it is more believable and acceptable.

You may tell others about what you have, but because they can't see it they'll tend to ignore or forget it unless reminded. They assume you have a life similar to theirs, so they may respond to you or ask you to do things you're unable to do. Once again you have to share what your limitations are. These may be received well or you may be pressured to just "give it a try" because "you'll feel better by trying." Because of a permanent foot injury, I (Norm) usually sit during the first 15 minutes of praise singing in the worship service I attend because the hard floor aggravates my injury. I'm sure some wonder, "Why isn't he participating more?" I could invest my energy wondering what they're thinking or tell myself, "It really shouldn't matter since they're unaware of my condition. And besides I'll never know if someone is really wondering about it."

The problem is that the expressions on the faces of those around you often tell more about their reactions than their words. They might not appear as compassionate and caring, especially if they've never had an invisible illness. It's the old adage, "You look healthy, so what's your problem?" One of the reasons for telling others is to prevent them from making assumptions about what is wrong with you. If there are some symptoms that are becoming more obvious, such as falling asleep at your desk, being absent, being late for work, wearing sunglasses inside, or having to go to the restroom frequently, these tend to lead to speculation.

Thinking through what you want to share and how to do so will help. Here are some possible scenarios:

> "I wanted you to know why I haven't been here as much as usual. I have an illness called fibromyalgia. It's hard for me to spell it, let alone describe the disease and what it's like living with it. Some days are better than others and if you ask how I'm doing you'll probably get different answers depending on the day. It's not contagious so you can relax on that score. I have some pamphlets that describe my condition if you'd like additional information. I would appreciate your prayers for strength."

> "I struggle with depression, so there are some days when you talk with me that I may appear as if the light's out…but I'm still here, I promise. This is something I'm learning to adjust to. It's caused by a chemical imbalance in my brain."[12]

One of the best approaches to sharing is planning the disclosure so you can protect yourself, others, and relationships. Again who, what, and how are the questions. The phrase "selective informing" is a process many employ. Sometimes there's a tendency to go overboard in softening the news for others. The negative aspects of the illness are usually downplayed. For some this seems to make it easier for the one who has the chronic illness. Sometimes it's done in a very factual informational manner, the lack of emotions making it easier to share. But both these approaches can leave questions in the minds of those hearing the news. Many focus on creating the "right" kind of setting in which to share.

Sharing invites people into your life so they can be involved with you by caring, supporting, helping, and praying. Yes, be selective in what you say, but also be truthful about the diagnosis and prognosis. The deeper the relationship, the greater the sharing depth. Knowing what to share takes wisdom and discernment on your part. You may want involvement and support from some, whereas with others you just want them to know.[13] Just as this is a crisis and a shock to you, so it will be for those who are closest to you. Let them have "process time." Be aware of your expectations for them. If they go unfulfilled, your relationships may be affected.

The following questions are designed to help you identify people in your life who might assist in your journey by being a supportive network.

- Who is the encourager in your life when you are struggling? Who would you like it to be?

- Who is the person you turn to for laughter and closeness? Who would you like it to be?

- Who stands by to help you move forward? Who would you like this to be?

- Who listens to your dreams? Who will help you create some dreams?

- Who will listen to you during your worst times? Who would you like it to be?

- Who do you share your spiritual life with? Who would you like it to be?

- When you need to run an errand or go shopping, who can you depend on to assist? Who would you like to have help you?

- Who do you go to when you're hurting? Who else is there that you could invite into your life to help you?

- Who helps you grow and learn in new areas? Who would you like it to be?

- Who do you feel safest with, and who supports you the most?

- Who are the people or groups that pray for you regularly? What support groups are available?

One of your tasks will be to monitor and modify your expectations of others when necessary. For one thing, friends or family are not mind readers. Unless you let them know what you're thinking and feeling, they won't know how to respond. You most likely won't be fully understood by others, and you really don't need 100 percent understanding from everyone. You need to accept that everyone will be different. Not everyone is good for everything. But family and friends can be counted on for various levels of help and understanding.

So how do you respond to the question, "How are you?" This is especially difficult when you know some people ask and really don't care in the least. You don't want to be seen as sick or as a complainer, so it's easy not to be honest by withholding details or avoiding the question. Don't let others—and what you think they feel—control your response. A positive way to respond when asked is to assume the person is sincere and to give an honest answer:

- "At the moment I feel..."
- "I may look all right, but I feel like a bulldozer ran over me."
- "Every day ranges from good to bad."
- "On a scale of 0 to 10 right now, I'm at a three."
- "My outside looks good, but inside I hurt."
- "Some days have been pretty good, but today is not one of them."

Chronic illness is a difficult road to travel. It's even more difficult when we experience it alone. If possible, engage others to walk with you in a supportive manner. This will take energy and effort that you may believe you don't have, but it's worth trying. Enlist support. Make a list of those you want or need to be your encouragers. Each day pray for God to work in their lives to strengthen them as well as touch their heart to reach out to you in a compassionate way.

Recommended Reading

We encourage you to read more about this subject. We recommend the following books. Some are written from a Christian perspective, while others are not.

Dawn, Marva. *Being Well When We're Ill.* Minneapolis: Augsburg Fortress, 2008.

Rosen, Michael, M.D., and Mehmet C. Oz, M.D. *You, the Smart Patient.* New York: Free Press, 2006.

Salves, Julie, M.D., *Chronic Pain and the Family.* Cambridge: Harvard University Press, 2004.

4

Your Family

Chronic illness is a family affair. Every person in the group is affected in some way. Too often some family members turn out to be sources of pressure and distress rather than support. That's because it's difficult for many of them due to the ongoing nature of long-term illness.

What is it like for family members? Most don't know what to say or do. Some may smother you with help, violate your boundaries, or add to your discomfort in some way. If you get too much attention, other family members may be resentful because they feel neglected. Some may ignore you. Others may feel your illness upsets the family balance. It's natural for family to want you to "be the way you used to be." Some may actually say this to you! Keep in mind others may be struggling with two common responses—guilt and feelings of potential obligation.

When one person in a family has a chronic illness, other members are thrust into a variety of new roles—including detective. Their world has also been changed. Now they look at you through different filters. They're looking for signs of pain, discomfort, improvement, and healing. You may not be comfortable with this change...or you may welcome it.

When you enter into the world of chronic illness and its accompanying grief, you become aware of how difficult and awkward it is for family and friends to express their concern. People usually don't know what to say or do since they decide how you're feeling through their own experiences with illness. They frequently don't fully understand and could come across as judgmental. You may be wounded or avoided, and this compounds your suffering. One of the best descriptions of this problem is in the book *Suffering and the Sovereignty of God:*

> People who love you often focus exclusively on "the problem." They ask about "the problem." They pray that God would solve "the problem." They offer advice for solving "the problem." They care for you! These are well-meaning attempts to be helpful. But the effect can become unkind. For example, many significant sufferings have no remedy until the day when all tears are wiped away. Your disease or disability is incurable.
>
> Other people are often clumsy and uncomprehending about the most important things, while pouring energy and love into solving what is unsolvable.
>
> This double suffering commonly occurs when a health problem eludes diagnosis and cure. Jesus met a woman who "had a hemorrhage for twelve years, and had endured much at the hands of many physicians, and had spent all that she had, and was not helped at all, but rather had grown worse" (Mark 5:25-26 NASB). Her story has a decidedly contemporary ring! Bleeding was a real medical problem. But attempts to help multiplied her misery. The subsequent two thousand years have not eliminated the phenomenon: faulty diagnoses, misguided treatments, negative side effects, contradictory advice, huge waste of time and money, false hopes repeatedly dashed, false fears pointlessly rehearsed, no plausible explanation forthcoming, blaming the victim, and declining sympathy as compassion fatigue sets in for would-be helpers! The woman was sick; other people made it worse.[1]

Think about your family. Who understands you and your illness the best? Who understands it the least? Which of their questions help you? What are the questions you hate to hear? Family members often have unasked questions that should be addressed. The ideal would be to sit down as a family and discuss them. Perhaps you or another family member might introduce the discussion by asking, "Have you been wondering" questions:

- "Why did she get this?"
- "Is this genetic? Can I get this too?"
- "Why her and not me?"
- "Has anyone else in our family ever had this?"
- "What can I do to help?"
- "What if the money runs out? I can't help."

Families are so prone to playing the blame game. The ones we love the most we often hurt the most. Self-doubt, shame, self-blame, and other blames are toxic responses. Chronic illness is dissimilar to someone experiencing a broken arm, a burned face, or having a crippling disease that limits mobility. The effects of these conditions are visible, and others are aware and can respond with compassion and sensitivity. In chronic illness, the pain and illness are real, but in so many cases invisible. Others often soon forget about it and fail to be supportive.

Chronic illness is similar to a natural disaster but without the fanfare of the media. We see the visible effects of a hurricane or tornado, but this time the house remains in place and the residents are the victims.[2]

As the person in pain, look at the expectations *you* have of each family member. Are they realistic? Can others give what you want? Let them know what you need…and do it with clarity. No one is a mind reader. Keep others abreast of how you're doing and whether it's a good day or a bad day. Let them know the steps you're taking to improve your quality of life. Don't be hesitant to talk about your illness and what you are learning about it.[3]

In an effort to be helpful, family members may offer unsolicited comments and advice:

- "You need to get a new doctor."
- "I heard that your doctor really misdiagnosed…"
- "I just heard of a new medicine that you've got to try."
- "Don't take that supplement. I heard it causes cancer."
- "You need to take that supplement. I heard it cures what you have."

- "This new diet could change your life."

- "Don't think about it."

- "Have you gone for healing prayer?"

- "Have you thought of seeing a counselor? A lot of this could be in your head."

It's easy to become irritated with all the well-meaning but unhelpful suggestions thrown at you. One of the best ways to respond is to simply say, "Thank you. I'll consider that" or "I may look into that." Then change the subject and move on.

If you're a parent, keep your children aware of your journey. Each child will respond differently. And just because children don't say anything or ask questions doesn't mean they're not thinking about it. Often, as in grief situations, children are left out of the equation. Young children may experience fear over their needs not being met, a sense of helplessness at not being able to do anything about what is happening, and perhaps feel they may have caused the problem. Some of their fears may come out as anger or acting out.[4]

Family Roles

Most family members can be identified by three different responses. Some may be *doers,* who use their anxiety to move into action. You'll see them taking control. They may gather information, protect you, and do whatever needs to be done.

Some become *detectives.* They're constantly looking for indications of the illness or discomfort. Their role may not be appreciated at times and seem intrusive.

Others are *retreaters.* They're overwhelmed by the illness and either do nothing or distance themselves. They need to process their thoughts and feelings. A common fear is, "I might get this as well."[5]

Other family roles may be affected also. How has your illness changed the dynamics in your family? Here's a chart to help you evaluate your situation.

Family Roles	Stayed the Same	Who Changed?
Assigner of household chores		
Breadwinner		
Confidant		
Cook		
Disciplinarian		
Doctor/nurse/veterinarian		
Financial decision maker		
Gardener		
Handyman		
Homework supervisor		
Housekeeper		
Instructor		
Liaison with school		
Link to extended family		
Martyr		
Nurturer		
Pusher for church attendance		
Rescuer		
Scapegoat		
Shopper		
Social director		
Victim[6]		

With chronic illness, the time you have with family will need to be shifted from quantity to quality since there will be many "time thieves" that come into your life. Your relationships will change since you're not your "old self." Instead of making polite requests you may bark out orders and then berate yourself afterward. Or perhaps it's hard to ask for help since you were used to being the caregiver. Maybe you're not getting the attention or help you need and resentment is building. Do you want to be like you used to be so much that you are wearing a "normal mask"? If so, others have no way of knowing how bad you feel. Once again the thoughts you have affects how you react. You may conduct a mental battle over "should I bother them with this? I've been such a bother already. I think they're getting weary." But honesty and openness are good policies. The best suggestions we've found for adjusting to living well with chronic illness and pain in a family come from *The Pain Survival Guide*, "Guidelines for Improving Communication Within a Family":

- Tell others respectfully what you can and cannot do.

- Inform them that the severity of your pain varies, and [the pain] may never be completely gone.

- Tell them in a friendly way what kind of help you hope to receive and why.

- Tell them when they are helping! Praise wins over blame every time.

- Do not be afraid to tell people when things are a bit better or a bit worse.

- If at all possible, try to be positive...despite the pain. A pleasant disposition can sometimes decrease pain at the same time it brings others closer to you.

- Ask for understanding with regard to your difficult feelings about the pain and its consequences. Give an honest answer to the question "How are you feeling?" Then show interest by inquiring as to how the other person is doing.

- Talk to others regularly, not just when your pain is most intense.

- Do not have important discussions, make rash statements, or make important decisions when your pain is at its worst.

- Do not use body language alone to indirectly communicate pain. Be direct and honest in telling people how you are feeling. Encourage others to express their feelings and to discuss them with you.

- Do not feel guilty if the pain has a negative influence on your moods. This is normal. Try not to take things out on other people, however.

- Work on accepting your present limitations as much as possible while making efforts to improve. This will involve what you say to yourself about your limitations. A "this is what I'm able to do at this time and that's all right" can be helpful.

- Do not take the other person's mildly negative behavior personally. Others' moods most often reflect their own personality or concerns.[7]

Friendships are also impacted. The energy it takes to maintain them is often not there. You may be limited in what you can do and when. Others may withdraw but so might you. They, like family members, won't know how to respond. It may be difficult to make new friends, but you may develop a circle of friends who are also struggling with chronic illness so they can relate to where you are. There's also the possibility that you may have more time for friends because of being unable to work.

The more you accept your condition the easier it is for those around you to accept it. And the more everyone understands your limitations and capabilities the easier it will be. But also maintain your boundaries regarding who is in charge. Janice said:

> I shared with my husband and two teens that I knew they were just looking out for me when we go out to eat. But it's better for me to ask these questions of myself than to be hammered by others. "What effect will it have on me?" "Is there too much sugar in this?" "Is this dessert all right?" I feel better about myself and my abilities when I can voice the questions myself.

Because you can't keep your illness from affecting your family, they will also hurt in their own ways. They too can become despondent because what they knew is no longer viable. Your family has "a front row seat at a home movie they never wanted to see. You are the reluctant center of attention, watching them watch you."[8] Your relationships change, albeit sometimes subtly. Do any of these sound familiar? And do these statements build a relationship or erode it?

- "I know I said I would clean out the garage today, but my legs were bad. I just didn't get to it. I promise I'll try tomorrow."

- "Why do you kids always start to pick at one another when I'm tired?"

- "John, I'm tired too. I have to put up with your illness, so you'll have to put up with my crabbiness."

- "I'm sick of trying to be heroic. I'm no angel of mercy."

- "Dr. Thompson says I'd better get a walker. He told me I might fall because my legs are getting so weak. I'm scared, honey. And I'm ashamed because you're embarrassed for me."

- "What do you mean we can't go? You promised me, didn't you? Your stupid illness gets in the way of everything."

- "I wish I'd never heard of lupus. It's ruined all our plans for the future."

- "I hate this illness. Everything I ever planned for myself is ruined. Why don't you go out and have some fun? There's no reason both of us have to sit on the sidelines."

- "Stop crying, you big baby. All you ever do is complain."

- "Look, I'm sorry. I thought you would be too tired to go. It was an honest mistake. You know I try to include you."

- "I see you broke another dish today. Maybe we should invest in a company that makes paper plates so we can pay some of these bills."[9]

The conversations you have with family members need to be open and honest. This may be painful and disheartening at times, but it's necessary and even healing.

Your Couplehood

Questions exist in the minds of both spouses. "When will I get well again?" "When will you get well again?" With chronic illness you can never say, "This is for certain." Life may not have the predictability it used to have. Sudden change becomes the norm. These issues need to be discussed. Talk and listen to your spouse about everything, including the fears and struggles that threaten to overwhelm you.

Financial stress has always played a significant part in marital relationships. Now it could be a constant worry with little opportunity to move ahead. If there's a job loss coupled with medical bills, there is less income and an increase of stress, which negatively impacts the illness.

One of the main disruptions at this time is the loss of emotional balance. When a significant illness occurs, couples can draw closer together and function as a team or they can fragment. Sometimes present conflicts are put on hold since the severity of the illness may take precedence. Grief and loss quickly become companions and, unfortunately, many spouses respond differently to loss than their partners. Few people understand the process of grief and the normalcy of their feelings, so their responses often include fear or they get stuck in the anger phase. Anger takes up residence, which can be especially destructive because it pushes a couple apart rather than draws them together. Anger at the illness, the symptoms, the diagnosis, the life change may be directed toward each other.

What About Intimacy?

The effect of chronic illness on your marriage is tied into the frequency and intensity of the illness as well as the degree of disability. If a spouse has periodic bouts with pain, there's a different impact on the marriage than a spouse with severe and constant pain. Each person handles illness by coping in different ways.

Chronic illness often encroaches into the life of a couple over a several year span. Or sometimes it's an overnight invasion. By definition, most chronic illnesses have no cure and so from this point on plans change, daily routines are derailed, finances are drained, and emotions are put to the test.[10]

Chronic illness brings a number of common bedfellows. *Low self-esteem* is primary. "I'm a burden on my spouse." *Guilt* occurs because "I can't contribute anymore." *Isolation* and *loneliness* soon arrive because "everybody else can get out, and I'm left alone so much of the time." *Worry* comes in easy especially regarding money and not being able to contribute. And *frustration* grows steadily since the rest of the world is moving on and "I'm trapped inside this diseased body with relentless pain and fatigue."

Thus the doubts come to reside, especially about God and His presence and concern.[11] It's easy for despondency to take up permanent residence.

If you're married, do you remember your wedding vows? There is a part in most vows that we all give lip service to and never imagine that it could happen to us...or at least not until we're in our nineties: "In sickness or in health." No one signs up for a chronic illness siege.

Imagine you've been married for 20 years. You're both employed, your two children are doing well, most of the bills are paid, and you're happy with one another. Enter chronic illness symptoms. Then enter the chronic illness diagnosis. Whether the realization is gradual or sudden, the diagnosis shatters your life as a couple.

As if your own feelings aren't enough to deal with, you have to deal with your spouse's reactions too. Many couples feel as if they've received two separate diagnoses, and in a way they have. Grief separates even the most compatible partners because, simply put, it's pain—pain that we must work through alone before we can reach out to our partners.[12]

In most marriages roles change over time and usually because the couple agrees to restructure the marital responsibilities and tasks. But when chronic illness hits a spouse, the roles can change slowly or suddenly without the consent of either partner. Sometimes the changes are a slow erosion that isn't noticeable on a day-by-day basis. The more disabled a spouse becomes, the more devastating it is. The balance of the relationship is thrown into disarray. The spouse with chronic illness can't do as much as before because of his (or her) condition, the pain, the loss of energy from the disease and possible side effects of medication. The "well" spouse now has more work to do at home and may have to increase hours at work for additional finances. And who is available to help out with parenting tasks?

The ill person struggles. It's difficult to live with someone who is losing or has lost the quality of life previously enjoyed. Often the healthy spouse is full of mixed emotions. It's difficult to admit his feelings, especially to the partner. And the well spouse feels guilt and remorse over feelings such as anger or resentment that come but aren't socially acceptable. One spouse said:

> Living with a loved one's illness is tragedy enough, but not being able to talk about it is a double tragedy. We make a bad situation

worse when we can't share the truth about it, a conspiracy of silence surrounds us because our reality differs so dramatically from public perception.[13]

The spouses of chronically ill people soon become somewhat invisible. They're overlooked by the medical profession. To them, it's the one with the illness who's important. Rarely are spouses asked, "How are you doing with this disease?" At the same time though, the spouse could also experience the "Plaster Saint Syndrome." It's a form of hero worship. He hears, "Oh, you're so good to her. You must love her so much" or she hears, "I could never do what you do. He's so lucky to have you."[14]

Sex becomes a major issue when your body hurts. Intimacy may be the last thing on your mind, yet you want to meet your spouse's needs. If you're a woman, you may wonder what your spouse is thinking and how long he can tolerate this situation.

Pain can limit sexual activity. If you're experiencing pain you may be afraid of increasing the discomfort, and your spouse may be afraid of inflicting more pain. Sexual interest and ability may diminish because of the disease, depression, and side effects of medication. Emotional responses such as anger, anxiety, or guilt play a part as well.[15]

If your sexual relationship isn't what it was (and perhaps never will be again), guilt may accumulate. It weighs on your mind that this isn't a satisfying situation. Once again you need to give your mate clear instructions on what is good for you and what isn't, what you can tolerate and what you cannot. Let him (or her) know what type of touching is helpful and what isn't.

Chronic illness is no respecter of personal boundaries. What happens because of the responses of others can influence the illness. One of the fears ill persons have is abandonment by their partners. Some people push their partners away, their fear becoming a self-fulfilling prophecy. Shoving a loved one away heads off the hurt of possibly being rejected. The well spouse struggles with, "Should I approach my partner sexually or not?"

Chronic illness can drive a couple together or create a wedge between them. Illness carries a byproduct called "change" which generates stress, which contributes to the destruction of relationships. It doesn't have to, but too often does. Changes in your marriage will happen, but you and your spouse can be in charge of them. If you can anticipate what they might be, determine what you would like to change. Anticipate the effects or fallout, and develop a new "normal" for your life and your couplehood so your marriage can become better. Just as a child disrupts a couple's "twosome" and turns it into a triangle (mother, father, and child), so chronic illness creates a new and awkward triangle—you, your spouse, and *it!*

The loss of the way "the relationship used to be" is hard on both spouses for different reasons. Coupled with the anger is the sadness and depression. The exhaustion, which both experience, unfortunately creates a scenario in which there is even less emotional control.

People with chronic illnesses can become angry at their spouses for doing too little…or for doing too much. The well spouses may not believe their partners' conditions are as bad as they really are. Both spouses live in constant fear of the future and what it may bring.

Studies indicate that 25 to 65 percent of those in relationships that include a chronic pain component have a decrease in marital satisfaction. Most of the time it's the well spouse who voices dissatisfaction. As many as 75 percent of the couples end their marriages. Some people choose to stay in a bad marriage because "Who else would want me in my condition?"[16] But your marriage doesn't have to be part of those negative statistics!

If you and your spouse work together to redefine and reshape your marriage, there is hope. This takes honest sharing and discussion. If there is ever an occasion for seeing a marriage counselor, this is the time. A third party who is knowledgeable about chronic illness' effects in a couple's life can assist your marriage in moving forward rather than deteriorating. You'll work on these skills and more:

- looking at what's working in your marriage rather than what isn't

- looking at what's frustrating you in your marriage and come up with two or three possible solutions

- discovering different ways to respond to each other

- discussing the responses each of you would like to see

Your marriage can not only survive, but it can grow in positive ways if you adjust and stay flexible. We'll talk more about coping with the changes and losses in a later chaper.

Chronic illness is not a journey you or your spouse or your family signed up for. "In sickness and in health" has become a reality. But it doesn't have to be just a time of dismay and disappointment. It can also be a time of growth and the realization of an even deeper commitment and love.

Chronic illness is a tremendous challenge for any family. Again, in the midst of the disruption and pain there is potential for individual and family growth.

How can any positives or any growth occur in the wake of chronic pain? In the midst of everything you feel and experience, if you turn to the One who can make something happen out of the chaos—to the presence of Christ with you, hope will prevail! Connect daily with Christ, reflecting on these verses from God's Word that speak of hope and strength:

> Not only so, but we also rejoice in our sufferings, because we know that suffering produces perseverance; perseverance, character; and character, hope (Romans 5:3-4).

> Fill up and complete my joy by living in harmony and being of the same mind and one purpose, having the same love, being in full accord and of one harmonious mind and intention (Philippians 2:2 AMP).

Recommended Reading

We encourage you to read the following books. Some are written from a Christian perspective, while others are not.

Dawn, Marva. *Being Well When We're Ill.* Minneapolis: Augsburg Fortress, 2008.

McGonigle, Chris, Ph.D., *Surviving Your Spouse's Chronic Illness.* New York: Henry Holt & Company, 1999.

5

The Power *of* Pain

Any discussion of chronic illness would be incomplete without covering the difficult…and even harsh…reality that many people suffer from chronic pain. From all-over aches to debilitating pain, people who suffer this way confront special challenges and questions, including wondering why a loving God would put them through such trials.

If chronic pain is part of your world or the world of someone close to you, there are ways to cope with the situation that can help mitigate the suffering.

The Constant Struggle

Pain? Let me tell you. It's constant.

It's so abnormal to have a time when it's not hurting. When you do, it's almost like you don't even realize what it's like not to have pain. And incapacitating fatigue goes right in there, along with depression too. What makes it worse is other people don't understand. They don't get it. They don't get that you feel bad every day of your life.

What is it like to be in constant pain?

It's there every moment. It's rare that I have half an hour free from pain or even 15 minutes, and the pain is in multiple areas too. If it's not my lower back, it's my neck, or if my neck gets a little better, it's my head or my back again. And when one area

71

clears up, something else starts to hurt. I wonder if it's not in degrees—yes—everything is there hurting all the time. It's just in degrees as to which one is the worst, and when one is really bad, it overshadows the others. When I have a migraine headache, my back doesn't seem to hurt as much. But when the migraine goes away, my back hurts worse. I'm never free.

And it's not an anticipation that something else is going to hurt. It's not an attitude of "Oh, now what?" No, it's reality. Unfortunately, other people tend to think I'm anticipating it. They say, "Oh you've had it before so you just think it's going to come back." I don't until it hits me.

Generally these things never go away. It's constant. I'm in constant pain to one degree or another. A lot of times it's multiple areas. If someone asks, "What are you going to do now?" I don't know for sure. It all depends. I have good intentions and plans for what I want to get done, but it all depends on my body. Sometimes I put pressure on myself and allow myself several days of being sick and then I say, "Okay, by this time you need to get up and accomplish this and that." I put pressure on myself to do what I'm not able to do. It's a big deal just to run an errand or change the sheets on my bed. It all hurts. And because my condition can't be seen, it doesn't elicit the care and understanding one would receive with a visible illness.

When a person has a chronic illness and comes down with a cold or the flu or bronchitis, it takes much longer to recover than the person who doesn't have a chronic illness. Others tell me, "Oh, that only took me five days to get over," but it could take me twice as long. People don't understand why, and they think I'm malingering. My body doesn't heal like a normal body. Recovery is prolonged. I actually have a malfunctioning immune system. It doesn't fight off the right things. Instead it says, "Go *attack* the joints or the muscles." It's supposed to protect and fight off disease and illness; instead, it attacks and destroys my body.

The threat of sudden, excruciating pain when you have a chronic illness can determine how you live your life. Many chronic pain sufferers have given up on expecting to feel good ever. And when they do have good days, it's like gifts from heaven. One woman said, "My illness is best described as terroristic. I have periods of good health, but they can be disrupted at any time with no warning." This physical pain incurs mental pain as well. Many have said they tend to feel ashamed or guilty when their illnesses take turns for the worse. Why? Because of the tendency to believe, "I got worse; therefore, I must have done something wrong." One woman describes her experience this way:

> The worst pain I know is all consuming. It evades other physical sensations and demands complete concentration. It creates a vacuum at the core that cannot be filled by any other emotions than hopelessness, helplessness, fear—the components of despair. Pain is extremely isolating. No one else can imagine or recall pain and feel it with the same intensity. While it lasts, it is all mine. It is like being enshrouded in my own body, unable to peer out, unable to feel anything but the body's immediate sensations.[1]

Yet another describes her daily struggle with pain:

> When people say, "I'm surprised you're not feeling better," it's like a convicting thing toward me because I feel convicted already. In our bodies it just takes longer because the immune system is messed up.
>
> When I wake up I feel so bad, but I think I have so much to do I need to get up and do it. But if I do, it will make me feel worse. I put pressure on myself because I feel there's something wrong with me. When someone else gets a cold they can get up and get over it. In 5 or 7 days they're back to normal. Why not me?
>
> What helped me so much this morning when I woke up, instead of just talking to myself about it, I began talking to God. I also began reading *Praying God's Word* because if my negative thoughts stay in my head and keep going around and around up there, it's not going to get any better. Then I get down and depressed. When other people don't understand, I feel damaged or faulty...and in reality I am. I have a damaged immune system. I'm learning to accept it, but it's still frustrating because I'd like to get up and go out. So, who or what do I listen to then?

My body or my "shoulds" or what I want to do? Sometimes it will be a compromise.

This does set a person up mentally for a different viewpoint. Instead of doing three things, I choose one and try not to feel bad about it. But how do I *not* feel bad about it? How do I not feel guilty? How do I not feel bad that what I want doesn't get done?

Pain has the power to dominate life. It's an attention grabber that can override whatever else is going on in your life. Pain interferes with sleep, exercise, eating, sexual activity, the ability to work, and interfacing with others. It undermines every aspect of your life. It goes hand in hand with a deteriorating life. Dr. Ira Byock graphically described the experience:

> As a physician I have seen the devastating effects that physical pain can have on people's lives. Acute pain, at least, sometimes protects us. We instantly remove our hand from a hot stove and remember to check before putting it there again. In contrast, chronic pain has no biological purpose. It can make proud, productive people feel useless and isolated. Whether it is daily migraines or relentless back pain, physical suffering captures a person's attention and doesn't let go. When you hurt, that's all you know. It leaves no room to enjoy life. Pain turns people inward and distorts their perceptions.
>
> Imagine what it would be like to have a stone in one shoe that you could not remove. With each step, you would feel a jabbing pain. You would hop or walk on tiptoe. You would learn to avoid certain streets or buildings that didn't accommodate your altered gait. This may seem a trivial example, but notice how one small stone affects you. No more tennis or bowling. No treadmill or StairMaster. No walking for pleasure. No dancing. You would have to admit the extent to which the chronic pain and accompanying physical limitations had changed your life and colored your perception of the world.[2]

Jeremiah the prophet described how so many feel:

Why has my pain been perpetual, and my wound incurable,
refusing to be healed? (Jeremiah 15:18 NASB).

You too wonder why God allows the pain to be inescapable. And you're
not alone in your pain. Between 15 and 20 percent of those in our country
live with chronic pain, with less than half getting adequate care.[3]

None of us want pain and none of us like pain. How have you lived
with it? How does anyone live with it? Especially when relief is elusive.
Only you are aware of the extent of your pain. Pain descriptions vary:

- "It's a constant toothache, although it's in all of my body."

- "It's like I've had the flu for the past three years and there's no
  relief."

- "For me, it's always there, but in the evening it's so intense I
  can't even move."

And so you try and try again to gain relief whether through medication, special postures and meditation, a special bed, acupuncture, nutritional supplements, EMDR, massage, hypnosis, cognitive behavior, and
so forth. What can you do? You can share with your doctors the extent
of your pain. Describe it in terms that register with doctors, such as a
scale of 0 to 10, zero meaning you're free of pain, whereas 10 means you're
immobilized by it.

Your Brain and Pain

Have you ever been told, "Your pain is all in your head?" Quite possibly, and if so you may have been offended or angry. Well, your pain is
"in your head," but probably not in the way the comment was originally
intended. Chronic pain isn't just a symptom of something else but a disease in its own right. When you're in pain, the emotion centers of your
brain are more active and so are your brain's sensory centers. You really
can't have pain without your brain being involved. But it's *not* a mental
illness. It's physical.

Chronic pain has more power than most realize because it disrupts
brain function. The problems it creates include sleep disturbances, depression, anxiety, and concentration issues. MRIs show that with no pain,

the brain has regions that reflect a state of equilibrium or rest. But for those with chronic pain, the area of the brain mostly associated with emotions never shuts off. It stays active and in time wears out the neurons that channel the connections to one another. If you could look into the brain of a person with chronic illness you might see a rewired brain that involves the hook ups and the areas related to emotion, pain, perception, and skin temperature.[4]

Other recent studies show that the brain receives pain messages from parts of the body through the spinal cord and nerve network. But it also undergoes changes in the nerve connections that may permanently strengthen its response to those signals.[5]

Dr. Martin Rossman, the author of *Guided Imagery for Self-Healing*, said, "While acute pain appears in areas of the brain that are connected to tissue damage, chronic pain lives in other areas of the brain—the prefrontal cortex and limbic system, which the brain uses for memories, especially emotional ones." In some cases "the pain lives on long past the time when the body tissues have healed." There is a reason why pain lingers. Repeated thoughts and emotions create nerve pathways in the brain. Chronic pain impulses travel along well-worn pathways.[6]

Your brain is there to help you. If you cut your finger, nerves immediately carry a signal to your brain that pinpoints the location of your injury and sounds the alarm to pull back from the cause to prevent additional injury. It then sensitizes an area around the cut to expand the area of protection. But it's not finished. It activates the body's pharmacy to produce its own set of painkillers, called endorphins. These provide temporary relief. But like any system, the brain can malfunction. In some cases, when the injury involves nerves, the wires for pain and everyday sensations can become "crossed." Instead of relief, there's constant pain.

Pain kills...your spirit, your drive, your hope, your relationships, and in some cases your life. Pain is a response. It can even be thought of as the body's way of expressing anger. If there's an injury, imagine your body complaining via pain. Pain creates suffering and interferes with life. If you ask, "How has pain intruded into my life?" what do the answers tell you?

There are different types of pain. The goal with acute pain is to diagnose the source and remove it. But with chronic pain the goals are to minimize the pain and maximize your functioning. Chronic pain is pain that has outlived its usefulness and is no longer beneficial. The pain is an unwanted and almost useless intrusion into your life.[7]

Your pain does have a purpose. It's a warning and, eventually, a request for help. Its message is, "Oh, oh! Something is wrong here." As it intensifies, it's saying, "Do something!" And when it's chronic, its message is, "I'm suffering."

The Social Impact of Pain

There's another kind of pain you may have to endure. Is your illness socially acceptable? That's really not a strange question. Acceptability of an illness as well as its symptoms varies. There are some illnesses that have a social stigma, which means you get even less support. No illness is really acceptable to society because if you're ill you can't contribute as much, you need special attention, you have special needs that often interfere with others' lives, and, what many don't like, you remind people that there is human weakness and your illness could happen to anyone.[8] (It's very much the same struggle when you've lost a loved one and you're in grief.)

When you have symptoms that aren't obvious or the illness isn't, people are naturally skeptical. That struggle was expressed well by Donaghue and Siegel:

> A high degree of social unacceptability of an illness can produce an extraordinary impact on the physiological well-being of a person. When we are ill we need the comfort of human sympathy and understanding. If a disease is deemed unacceptable, overtly or covertly, by society, its victims suffer the added burden of isolation and shame. They might even be dissuaded from seeking diagnosis and treatment.

> Coping with a chronic illness is challenging, but it is more tolerable when we can share our fear. The more socially unacceptable an illness, the less it is shared. Ironically, when we are scorned, distrusted, and rejected by others, we are prone to attack ourselves with the same attitudes.

> Every person who has an invisible chronic illness endures a

diagnostic process that is exasperating, terribly expensive and emotionally and physically painful. The ones who receive a clear diagnosis (the sooner the better) have the relative "comfort" of knowing what is causing their symptoms and what they must prepare to face. Others are left to confront the agonizing quandary of a vague diagnosis—or worse, no diagnosis at all.[9]

The inability to talk about your illness because of society's response creates additional stress and pain.

The Truth About Pain

Pain is very personal. We all experience it from a rose thorn in the finger to a throbbing toothache, from a pulled back muscle that radiates pain to a pinched nerve that strikes like a knife. Pain usually goes away over time and there is that wonderful sense of relief we so desire. But chronic pain is another animal indeed. It's constant and unrelenting. It interferes with daily living and continues past the normal time for healing. Some pain never goes away.

Chronic pain is real, but often the cause isn't obvious. For example, in up to 85 percent of those with back pain, doctors are unable to find a physical cause.[10] And when medical tests don't determine the cause, you may be told the pain isn't real, you're overreacting, or "it's in your head." Many illnesses don't "show up" as expected. There will also be times when you can't determine why or how you got the pain in the first place. One of the most unanswerable questions to be asked if you have a cold is, "Where did you get that cold?" If you knew, you would have avoided it! And usually you're not concerned "where" you contracted the sickness but rather what you can do to get over it. It's the same with chronic pain. What can you do to deal with it or manage it so you can get the most out of life?

There's an abundance of misinformation about pain, and unfortunately many believe it without question. Pain can be a sign of physical damage and injury but not always as some believe. It's not always reliable as to location and extent. One of the worst misbeliefs is that if you can't identify the cause, it must be imaginary. (It's too bad that others can't feel what you feel!)

If your chronic pain doesn't respond to a doctor's prescribed treatment, then some people believe the problem may not be that bad after all. And unless a doctor verifies that you have pain, some people—and even you—question whether it's real or as bad as you said. But *you're* the expert on the intensity of your pain, not anyone else. People aren't equipped to adequately measure another person's pain experience.

Medication and/or surgery are often the expected answer for every pain. These may help, but often they don't, and there may not be a cure-all for your condition.

An Answer to Pain

You may hear from the medical community that they have done all they can and now you have to learn to live with your problem. But there are other options. Very few doctors have had the opportunity to take specialized training in pain management. Believing there is nothing else to do will cripple your motivation and efforts and lead to despair and hopelessness. It's sad how many accept the belief that nothing more can be done and let this dominate their lives.[11] (See the alternative treatments listed in the back of this book.)

Pain isn't simple. In fact, it is quite complex, which is why a pain management team is helpful. In this way the problem can be addressed from different angles.

Your pain team needs a leader, a qualified person who can rule out underlying conditions, prescribe medication if necessary, and coordinate treatment. This is especially important when you're using alternative therapies so you can make sure they won't aggravate your condition or combine poorly with existing treatments. For this task, you'll want a conventionally licensed physician. It's best if you can find someone who actively practices integrative medicine or who is at least interested in it.[12]

Too many people with and without chronic pain have lived their lives looking backward, trying to discover "What happened?" or "What went wrong?" They're past-oriented instead of future-oriented or solution-focused. Life takes on a different flavor, even with pain, when you work on "How do I get a handle on my pain?" rather than "Where did this originate?" Being able to determine the cause isn't nearly as helpful as "What influences my pain?" And perhaps the most significant question is, "What can *I* do about my condition?" You need to take charge and not rely too much on others to make decisions for you. When it comes to managing your pain, it's really you who determines what to do, as well as taking the needed steps.[13]

One of the best steps you can take is to tell the story of your pain, including its history, to someone else—especially your doctor. Write your story down, for this can be beneficial in and of itself. As you write, you may see connections between changing circumstances, your treatments, and the amount of pain you've felt. Describe what your life was like before the pain, when it started, what you did about it, and what the pain has kept you from doing that you would like to do again.[14]

There are many words to describe pain. These adjectives may help you to be specific about your pain:

aching	itchy	spreading
agonizing	killing	squeezing
annoying	lancing	stabbing
blinding	miserable	stinging
cold	nagging	suffocating
cool	numb	taut
cramping	piercing	tearing
cruel	pinching	tender
crushing	pounding	throbbing
drawing	pressing	tight
dull	prickling	tingling
electrical	pulsing	tiring
exhausting	radiating	torturing
frightful	rigid	troublesome
gnawing	sharp	tugging
heavy	shooting	unbearable
hot	sickening	vicious
icy	smarting	wrenching[15]
intense	sore	

Let's continue with your history of your pain. This evaluation of your pain will be helpful, and you may want to use it as is or put it into another format to share with others to enlighten them about your current state.

Your Pain History

1. In the following list of activities, put a star by the ones you can still do. Add activities not listed that are important to you. Now go back and place a check by those you're unable to do because of your pain.

clean house	work in the garden
cook/bake	work on hobbies
go to the movies	work on the car
hold a job	worship
hunt or fish	•
play cards or board games	•
play sports (team or individual)	•
shop	•
visit with friends	•
walk in the park	•

2. After adding any activities that are important to you, circle the activities that have eased your pain in the past.

bath (warm)	rest
devotional reading	sleep
exercise	supportive friends
medication	•
prayer	•
relaxation	•

3. Circle the activities and circumstances that have made your pain worse in the past, including other things you've noticed. Also note what you've done to adjust.

arguments	sleep (poor)
cold	stress
depression	weather[16]
exercise	•
fatigue	•
heat	•

Another way of describing and evaluating your pain is by completing a detailed diary. By doing this, you may find new ways of responding. Keep this diary for days or even weeks, and share it with your pain management team. (See "A Pain Diary" in the back of this book.) We also recommend reading *The Chronic Pain Solution* by James N. Dillard, M.D., D.C., with Leigh Ann Hirschman.

Your Mental Anguish

Physical pain is bad enough in and of itself, but unfortunately it's intensified by the mental anguish that is also created. Sometimes your mental despair takes precedence over the physical. There are specific steps you can implement to take charge.

- *Identify your mental pain.* What feelings are you experiencing? Can you determine the cause for your feelings? Is it lack of rest or an overabundance of physical pain? What is contributing to your mental state? When you can answer these questions, you're closer to a solution.

- *Accept that you're in physical and mental pain.* What steps can you take to minimize it? Who can you share your feelings with? Describe how you're praying about this pain.

- *Accept and then release any feelings* that are not beneficial for you. Anger and fear are often at the heart of mental discomfort. We will discuss this more in the chapter on emotions.

- *Be sure to ask advice and feedback* from people who are objective. Often they can see what you can't.

- *Use humor and laughter* to get through the difficult time. It's a good way of taking a break from the heaviness of pain, loss, and grief.

- *Pray…and then pray some more…and enlist others to pray.* Ask for more strength, the perseverance you need, the change in your health that you desire, and the comfort that will make your situation bearable.

- *Change your scenery.* Just moving from one room to another can affect your attitude. Have someone rearrange your room. Bring in fresh flowers unless you have an allergy. Take steps to move your mind from despair to hope.

- *Reach out to help someone else.* I know this sounds crazy when you're feeling so bad, but when you give to others you get energized and feel a sense of purpose and meaning. Studies have shown that when we help someone through an act of kindness, we experience a physical benefit of increasing endorphin levels. If others are caring for you, find a way to do something for them as well.[17]

Getting sick is a time of turmoil and uncertainty. You don't know if you will always be sick. You believe you'll recover and get back to normal. Some symptoms come and go, as do possible diagnoses. The doctors diagnose but sometimes aren't sure. This is a time of searching, which often generates fears. Finally you may get a diagnosis.[18]

Being Sick

When George Burns reached the age of 90, he was asked what advice he would give to others who desired such longevity. His answer? Find a chronic illness and learn to live with it. The phase of "being sick" is not a sprint, but a long-distance journey. This race must be run with the determination of a highly trained athlete in order to successfully cope with the limitations of illness, the physical ups and downs, and the roadblocks common in the healthcare system.

The journey is challenging for everyone involved, not just you, the patient. Loved ones are also part of your team, and their need for support can be remarkably similar to yours. Teamwork, taking action, regaining control, and finding a balance—these are the necessary ingredients for making the transition from "getting sick" to "being sick."

So where do you begin? You must listen to your body, as well as to the advice of others. Then you must use the knowledge you gain to change your actions and bring balance to your life.[19]

Being sick has been described in many ways, one of which is "a war." It starts as a conflict that requires determination and skill. Who are you at war with though? You're fighting pain, fatigue, sometimes doctors and insurance companies, sometimes employees or employers, sometimes family and friends who question whether you're really ill because "you don't look sick." You're also battling yourself. The war you're fighting is to build a new life that contains illness but isn't defined by it. Winning this war means embracing the enemy. It involves accepting that you have a chronic illness.[20]

You'll find many helpful suggestions in this book on living with chronic illness. The following are guidelines to living well from a woman who was diagnosed with "undifferentiated connective tissue disease," as well as fibromyalgia and intestinal cystitis. (I [Norm] have added some explanatory text to help you.)

- *Put yourself first.* This may be contrary to your beliefs or the way you were raised. You need to take care of you or…well, you can imagine the results.

- *Never give up* no matter what you experience or how you feel.

- *Don't quit or become resigned* because you just don't have the energy. Continue to search for answers and solutions. Don't take a "no" or a closed door as a defeat, but see it as, "Well, I've looked into that and it wasn't the answer so I can cross it off the list and look elsewhere." Attitude is critical. It's similar to a fishing experience my wife, Joyce, and I (Norm) had a few years ago. We were in a boat fishing for trout at Lake Gregory. We had tried several spots on the lake without even the hint of a bite from a fish. As I pulled up the anchor several hours later, Joyce asked, "Oh, are we going in now?" I replied with, "Oh no. We'll just move to a new spot." "But we haven't caught a fish all morning," she said. My answer (which didn't go over well) was, "Yes, but at least we know where the fish aren't." It's the same principle here. Keep searching.

- *Know who you are now,* and let others know. The way you answer questions, especially, "How are you?" will be critical. If you're not doing well, say so. This is who you are at this time. Don't worry about being seen as a complainer. You seldom know what others really think about you, so why give that issue any of your precious energy? It's what you and God think about you that's important. You can say, "You know I have this chronic illness, and today is not a good day, so I appreciate your understanding if I'm a bit slow. Thank you."

- *Discover what works for you.* It may seem like you're on a continual search, like a prospector looking for a gold mine. Your doctor may have to use trial and error just as you do. If you have vague symptoms and unclear causes, the treatment may not be that clear either. Surviving is an ongoing process, not a one-time experience.

- *Make peace with your fatigue.* That will take some of the stress out of your life. We would all like to do what we were used to doing and love to do. But now you must do what you can and not do what you can't. And then thank God for what is and say goodbye to what isn't.

- *Living outside the box occasionally* will help your attitude. When you do something new, different, or something you used to do consistently, you're pushing and testing the boundaries of your illness. Who knows? You may experience something positive you never thought could occur.[21]

- *Figure out a way to help others.* What you are experiencing you would never wish on another person, but there are others who need to learn what you've discovered. Your experience can become a source of comfort and help to others. And when you give, you'll feel useful again. Scripture talks about this opportunity: "Praise be to the God and Father of our Lord

Jesus Christ, the Father of compassion and the God of all comfort, who comforts us in all our troubles, so that we can comfort those in any trouble with the comfort we ourselves have received from God. For just as the sufferings of Christ flow over into our lives, so also through Christ our comfort overflows" (2 Corinthians 1:3-5).

Recommended Reading

We encourage you to read more on this subject. In the following list, some books are written from a Christian perspective, while others are not.

Dawn, Marva. *Being Well When We're Ill.* Minneapolis: Augsburg Fortress, 2008.

Dillard, James, M.D., D.C., C.Ac., *Chronic Pain Solution—Your Personal Path to Pain Relief.* New York: Bantam Books, 2002.

Turk, Dennis C., Ph.D., and Frits Winter, Ph.D. *The Pain Survival Guide.* Washington, DC: American Psychological Association, 2005.

6

Dealing *with* Loss

L oss." It's a simple four-letter word that signifies one of our constant companions throughout life. But we don't talk about it very often. Like a silent conspiracy, we seem to have an unspoken agreement not to talk about what we can't do anymore. Yet with each loss comes the potential for positive change, growth, insights, understanding, and refinement. One reason could be that these hope-filled opportunities are realized or come in the future, and we fail to see that far ahead when we're in the midst of grief.

The losses of chronic illness are often hidden. Some of them can be retrieved, some partly recovered, while some are permanent. Although we tend to ignore the losses, the emotional experiences of them are planted in our hearts and minds and no eraser can remove them.

The majority of losses we experience are difficult to grieve over, especially chronic illness. Why? Because losses aren't usually recognized as such. In chronic illness, there's no body, no funeral, and no public shoulder to cry on. There is no traditional, socially sanctioned outlet for mourning when the losses aren't death related. Loss of physical functioning, relationships, and financial resources are not shared and mourned. There is no printed obituary, no "remains" laid to rest, no public gathering to cement the fact and focus love and support on the sufferers.

Trying to mourn loss when death isn't involved is a lonely wasteland, with vague beginnings and endings defined more often by the intangible dimensions of lost and found hope than by the perimeters of the crisis itself.[1]

We all live with fear, and the fear of loss is deeply ingrained within us. Every loss we experience, from early infancy on, becomes part of this pool of fear. When chronic illness strikes, our fear becomes reality.

When we think of loss, what usually comes to mind is death, a relationship breakup, a house destroyed, an auto accident, or something valuable stolen. But the losses in chronic illness, which may seem invisible or insignificant to an outsider, are momentous to the one experiencing them. When it's difficult to stand or comb our hair, sign our names legibly, climb stairs, or sit in regular chairs—those are major losses. Strength moving to weakness, independence moving to dependence, feeling sick rather than well soon define our lives. Physical losses nullify some hopes and dreams.

Is it the loss that throws us so much? Or could it be our perception or interpretation of what the loss means? We want to stop the decline, which we can't do, but we can change what the loss means to us. There is a choice! We're not talking a denial of the devastation but an acceptance of its effects and how to move on from here. Many of us measured our self-worth and identity by what we could do in a day. Now we need to find another guide. The old standards won't work anymore. And the old standard was never the one God used to value us anyway! As one woman said:

> As I confronted the fact that I had wrapped up my identity in things that I've physically done—the dancing, the drawing, dressing myself, or whatever—my previous investment in the physical doing began to melt away. And as it did, I discovered something beyond it. What I began to see was that my measure of worth did not need to be wrapped up in my actions or physical accomplishments. I saw that there clearly is a way that we participate in life that is quite beyond that. The breakthrough I experienced that evening was that as we give up our physical identification, we discover the spiritual. And this seems to happen even for those who, like me, never thought of themselves as spiritual before.
>
> In private, in meditation, in support groups, I have found little glimpses of the reality that lies beyond those measurements of

self-worth that no longer apply to my life. I know that my true identity cannot be found in my body or in my accomplishments in the external world; I am not my flesh and bones. I am a child of God, and God adores me. It is with this realization in mind that I have learned to cope with my worldly losses. My prayer has been, "May I become more radiant than my external self."[2]

What we're suggesting is not a one-time experience but something that needs to be revisited from time to time. The following questions are designed to help you understand the number of losses you've already experienced and their effects on your life and your family.

- At this moment in time, identify the loss or losses you're experiencing.

- How have these impacted your life?

Why not construct your own illness and loss timeline? You may find it very helpful. Jim's "Loss History" on the next page is a good illustration.

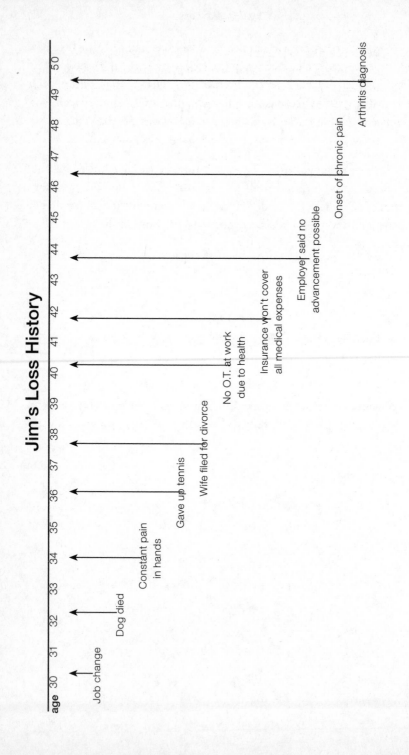

Jim's Loss History

age 30 31 32 33 34 35 36 37 38 39 40 41 42 43 44 45 46 47 48 49 50

Job change

Dog died

Constant pain
in hands

Gave up tennis

Wife filed for divorce

No O.T. at work
due to health

Insurance won't cover
all medical expenses

Employer said no
advancement possible

Onset of chronic pain

Arthritis diagnosis

Now, let's consider the impact each loss has had on your life. First look at the emotions or feelings in the following list. Take each loss and identify which emotions or feelings best describe your experience. These emotions are uninvited guests, but their intrusion is normal and their presence is temporary. Write the emotions by your timeline entries.

angry	feeling like a failure	numb
beaten	frightened	outraged
challenged	giddy	overwhelmed
compromised	handicapped	pain
crippled	happy	panicked
damaged	hopeless	relieved
defeated	hurt	self-hating
defective	inadequate	sickened
devastated	incapable	silly
disabled	incompetent	suicidal
disgusted	indecisive	susceptible
envious	inferior	vulnerable
exhausted	joyless	weak[3]
fearful	listless	
feeling inferior	melancholy	

The next step is to identify what you've learned from your losses up to this point. Remember, learning is an ongoing process. Some of the additional losses you may experience or have experienced may be:

ability to protect	energy	freedom
affection	equality	independence
autonomy	expectations of the future	innocence
body image		memory
cognitive function	faith	mental fog
competence	financial power	optimism

patience	self-esteem	shared responsibili-
physical function	self-image	ties
privacy	sense of control	social contact
resilience	sexual communica-	visibility[4]
security	tion	

Employment

For many, experiencing a chronic illness means the death of employment. And it is a death. It's not just the work itself that is taken away, but related pluses too. And many of those are attached to how we feel about ourselves—our self-esteem. We feel good about ourselves when we feel good about what we accomplish in our vocation.

For many, work is the hub of their social lives. At work you connect with others, build lasting friendships, and engage in social interaction. When you leave work because of chronic illness, these too tend to disappear.

Work has another meaning. It's an opportunity to express yourself. You can achieve, be creative, and even have new experiences. One man said, "When I couldn't work anymore, it wasn't just the pain of my illness. It was the feeling of being dried up inside. I stagnated." And for those who love to serve and help others, this avenue of caring is cut off and now *they* need to be served. This is very uncomfortable if your calling in life is to serve others.

For many, the loss of work is also the loss of lifelong dreams, and much of the substance of life is made up of dreams and desires. Dreams give you hope and inspiration, and it's not easy to see them die.

Few individuals understand the depth of loss that comes from not being able to work anymore. As one woman said, "Dying can't be any worse than losing your ability to work." Work is a valued role that has been taken away. And many people with chronic suffering have no possibility of returning, so this contributes to depression and loss of self-esteem.

Losing a job or being unable to do your work is like a final statement, a death knell in a way. "I'm someone who is chronically ill" hits home hard. The loss of your work is usually accompanied by and multiplied by other losses as well. If there isn't any hope of reentering the workforce, this situation can be even more difficult to accept. And, of course, job loss creates sacrifices for other family members as well. The loss of identity tied into work means you have to redefine yourself—and that's not easy. It can be overwhelming.[5]

Judith Viorst, in her book *Necessary Losses,* wrote about the idea of "shifting images," which is exactly what happens when a chronic illness invades your life:

> We mourn the loss of ourselves—of earlier definitions that our images of self depend upon. For the changes in our body redefine us. The events of our personal history redefine us. The ways that others perceive us redefine us. And at several points in our lives we will have to relinquish a former self-image and move on.[6]

When you're chronically ill, your losses are often magnified because of being singled out as sick and stigmatized. Your past seems to have been taken from you because the emphasis is on now. Many attempt to recapture their pasts, which is futile. They attempt to override their pain and continue to work as long as possible. This is partly an effort to maintain one's public identity: "See, it's me! I can still work in spite of what I have." Eventually though, work falls by the wayside.

What may help you is reshaping your life and your identity. Those who develop a strategy for redefining who and what they are usually move ahead.[7]

Along with missing work, the financial loss can also be overwhelming. Not only is there the loss of income, but you're experiencing additional medical expenses as well. This adds even more stress and pressure and usually demands a change in your lifestyle.

Then there are the losses of some family roles as well, from necessary tasks for day-to-day functioning to relationships. Often the roles related to nurturing and support experience the greatest amount of disruption. When a spouse is able to take over those roles, the family continues to function with less disruption.

The Loss of Some Intimacy

Chronic illness has another companion that may also bring two other losses—the loss of hope and the loss of sexual desire. You lose the awareness of your desirability and attractiveness, which affects your self-esteem. Sexual activity can begin to feel like a chore, like just another demand. You're also physically reluctant or unable to participate at times due to pain. Illness tries to cheat you out of so much in life. And your spouse may end up living as a "married widow or widower," sexually speaking. One author described the impact of chronic illness and losses upon a husband this way:

> Throughout their marriage, as his wife's conditions worsened, more responsibilities fell on him. He describes a "rolling grief" that living with a chronically ill spouse incurs. He didn't notice changes on a day-to-day basis, but when he stepped back and looked at how much had changed gradually—the jobs and tasks his wife used to do but couldn't, the number of plans or trips they'd cancelled, the decrease in their physical intimacy, the increased time he spent doing things for her—he was stricken by the magnitude of the losses for each of them. "Fairly early on I learned to set really low expectations for what we could and would do so I wouldn't get upset if plans fell through."[8]

How do you mourn the losses you both see daily, etched in your loved one's face? Dreams about children, career goals, retirement, travel—how can these losses be shared without damaging your relationship? If you and your partner can get in touch with where you are in your own grief cycle, and find a way to go beyond your individual pain to be mutually supportive, you will go on to restoration of yourselves individually and as a couple. Grief isn't just a one time event. It's recurring but the following description of a grief cycle will describe some of the common stages you may experience as well as what you may be thinking or feeling during each one. Some of your thoughts could be different. You may want to decide if you have experienced these stages as well as identify the thoughts and feelings you've experienced. A couple's cycle of grief looks something like this. Notice the progression. Perhaps you will find yourself traveling this path as well.

A Couple's Grief Cycle

Denial

Chronic illness sufferer: Maybe if I don't give in to my fatigue, it will go away.

Healthy spouse: I don't want to believe this is happening. Maybe in three months she'll be her old self.

Protest

Chronic illness sufferer: I feel betrayed by my own body. Where is God?

Healthy spouse: Darn it all! This shouldn't be happening to me...to us.

Chronic illness sufferer: Some days I feel guilty that I'm burdening my family by being sick.

Healthy spouse: How can I enjoy a good run when he can barely walk? First I feel guilty, then outraged!

Chronic illness sufferer: My energy is precious. And so is life!

Healthy spouse: Time is precious. Let's make the most of it.

Fear

Chronic illness sufferer: Fear, that's what I feel. What will happen to me in my old age?

Healthy spouse: The cold jaws of fear tell me that I am alone and responsible for the major efforts for this family. And this situation will go on and on.

Chronic illness sufferer: It scares me when I find myself thinking how they would be better off without me.

Healthy spouse: Some days I fantasize walking away from all this and starting out new somewhere. First I feel free, but then the guilt comes crashing down.

Chronic illness sufferer: It's embarrassing to feel and look so much older than I am.

Healthy spouse: Where do we belong? Most of our friends have gone away. My partner seems so old. I wonder how old I seem?

Ambivalence/Bargaining

Chronic illness sufferer: Just let me get these kids raised before I get much worse.

Healthy spouse: Just give us a few more good years. We have so much to do.

Sadness/Depression

Chronic illness sufferer: I think I was coping better before. What's wrong with me?

Healthy spouse: Sad, just sad, that's how I feel most of the time.

Chronic illness sufferer: Why get up in the morning? I just want to hide in the warm, safe bed.

Healthy spouse: I feel old before my time. My parents are dealing with the same things we are.

Chronic illness sufferer: It's lonely in my safe cocoon, yet I don't have the energy to get out.

Healthy spouse: Beat up and worn down, that's how I feel. Oh, to have time for myself...or just to rest!

Restoration

Chronic illness sufferer: If my body is going to be old, my spirit will be young.

Healthy spouse: This sure makes a person grow up in a hurry. I won't say I'd rather not have learned this way.

Chronic illness sufferer: I've changed a lot. I'm not sure I like the new me.

Healthy spouse: I've had to temper my impatience. I feel changed. I can't explain it.

Chronic illness sufferer: I have so much respect for my spouse. I didn't know my partner had such strength.

Healthy spouse: We're making it! There's a new mellowness to us that's come.

Chronic illness sufferer: The last relapse was something else. I hope this remission lasts a long time. There's lot's to do!

Healthy spouse: I'm getting familiar with the cycles now. Trust and faith that we'd get to this point kept me going.

Chronic illness sufferer: My energy is precious. And so is life!

Healthy spouse: Time is precious! Let's make the most of it.[9]

Grief Accumulates

Chronic illness and pain bring continual losses and grieving, whereas many other losses (including death) have some type of closure. The first indication of your life journey of losses is when the onset of symptoms hits and remains. You, your family, and your close friends will be stunned. Shock and disbelief can be expected. You make plans but soon learn you have to be open to adjusting them. For some, the acceptance of their illness comes quickly. But for others it's a slow realization, depending on the illness and how much they resist the diagnosis. And then, in addition to the illness itself, you're besieged by feelings and thoughts. The "Ball of Grief" has helped many identify and give voice to their emotions. Why not circle the ones you can relate to?

Grief: A Tangled Ball of Emotions

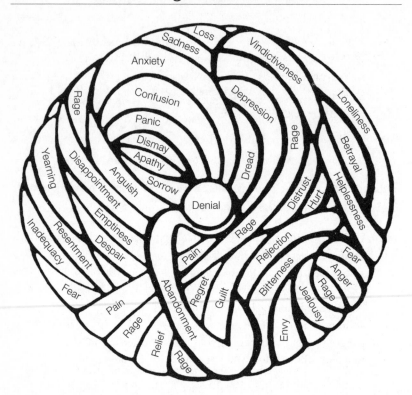

Part of you wants to do something and part of you wants to run away. And denial will be part of your life. Who wants to deal with chronic illness all the time? If you've experienced denial, you're normal. It happens because you're neither ready to handle the news of the illness nor can you grasp all the implications. You'll probably experience a mental numbness that follows an emotional wound. You may dismiss the news, rationalize it, or question whether it's true. This denial comes in a number of packages and gives you time to catch your emotional breath.

- There's the *denial of personal relevance:* "So what. I have a chronic illness. It's not a big deal. I can handle this."

- There's the *denial of urgency:* "It's all right. I have plenty of time, and this will take years to develop."

- There's the *denial of vulnerability:* "I've known others with this, and they seem to get along all right. To look at them, there's no problem."

- We also *deny our feelings:* "It's all right if it slows me down. I can do other things. This isn't that big of a deal."

- And then we may *deny the sources of our feelings:* "I have these strange sensations and I've been tired, but I know it's not because of the illness."

- We *deny information:* "They haven't proven anything yet. That's all speculation on their part."[10]

As denial subsides, anger creeps in as a protest. You feel betrayed:

> You may feel trapped in a failing body, humiliated by the extent of your inadequacies, surprised by your vulnerability, and angered and saddened by the loss of a youthfully responsive body. Perhaps you are heartsick over the threat to your spontaneity and at being treated unfairly by a demanding and far-from-benevolent culture. A part of you is searching for the "old me"; a part of you is struggling with cutting your losses and getting on with it, though it would help if you knew what "it" is going to be.
>
> Along with all of these feelings is the constant chatter in your head, much of it the voice of guilt: "Why didn't I take better care of myself? Will anyone ever love me again? What is wrong with me? Why am I this way? Why didn't I appreciate my body more when I was well?"[11]

Many move into a phase of bargaining. This too is a protest and a desire to get back to the way life and your body used to be:

> And then it hits—a dark cloud of depression. It's a time, a painful time, of assessing who you are now, that you've lost your future and are facing uncertainty. Out of this time acceptance can arrive. But it's important to remember your sense of loss and grief is ongoing. With the death of a loved one there is a pattern of grief that is completed and moving on to develop a new life. Yours will probably be a pattern of continual loss and

grief over and over again. You cycle through this, but you will learn through each experience as you learn to develop better and better coping skills.[12]

Constant loss can mean constant anger. All that changes is the level as it fluctuates. It's like a pot of liquid on the stove ready to erupt if someone turns up the heat. And it's not just your anger, but also that of your family members.

- You may be angry at yourself for not doing enough.

- You may be angry because of the change in lifestyle inflicted upon you.

- You may be angry over role changes that have to be made within your family.

- You may be angry for what is perceived to be a loss of control in your life.

- You may be angry that family and friends have gone back to their normal lives and aren't thinking about you as much.

- You may be angry that the rest of the world busies itself around you as though nothing has happened.

- You may be angry with God.

- You may have a combination of anger and depression, such as irritability, frustration, annoyance, and intolerance.

- You will feel some anger and guilt—or at least some manifestations of these emotions.

- You will have trouble thinking about memories, organizational tasks, intellectual processing, and making decisions.

- You may feel like you're going crazy.

- You may find yourself acting socially in ways that are different from before.

- You may find yourself having a number of physical reactions other than your illness.

- Others will have unrealistic expectations about you and may respond inappropriately to you.[13]

There are other losses that those who are healthy never dream about occurring. There is the fear and possibility of being rejected and labeled when others hear you have a chronic illness. Most of us want to be known for attributes other than an illness label. And people will respond differently so many avoid disclosing their illness in the hopes of avoiding yet another loss. We rely upon the generic phrase "I'm fine" to avoid sharing what we're really experiencing. We protect ourselves against further loss.

With losses there will be grief, which expresses basically three things:

- Through grief you express your feeling about your loss—and there will be a wide range.

- Through grief you express your protest at the loss as well as your desire to change what happened and have it not be true. You may begin to sound like David as he essentially cried out in the psalms, "How long is this going to go on? Won't this ever end?" (Psalm 13:1). This question of David's may be raised again and again throughout the day. "God, why have you forgotten me?" (42:9). "Are you going to forget me forever?" (13:1). You end up feeling neglected not just by others but by God. "How long will you hide your face from me?" (13:1). If you're like others you feel abandoned. David even questioned whether God was really God and you may have the same questions:

  – Will God ever show His favor on me again?

  – Has His love for me vanished?

  – Has His promise failed?

  – Has He forgotten to be merciful? (77:7-9).

- Protesting with questions is normal. You're not alone when you do.

- Through grief you express the effects you have experienced from the devastating impact of the loss.[14]

The overall purpose of grief is to bring you to the point of making necessary changes so you can live with the loss in a healthy way. You may not want to, but it's one of your choices. You begin with the question "Why did this happen to me?" and eventually move on to "How can I learn through this experience? How can I go on with my life?" When the "How?" question replaces the "Why?" question, you have started to live with the reality of the loss.[15] "Why" questions reflect a search for meaning and purpose in loss. "How?" questions reflect your searching for ways to adjust to the loss. Your eventual goal is to be able to say:

> This loss I've experienced is a crucial upset in my life. In fact, it is the worst thing that will ever happen to me. But is it the end of my life? No. I can still have a rich and fulfilling life. Grief has been my companion and has taught me much. I can use it to grow into a stronger person than I was before my loss.[16]

Mourning is the necessary process of returning back to life after we've been jolted from its road. It involves leaving behind what needs to be left behind, bringing along what needs to be brought along, and learning to distinguish between the two.[17] What do you have to do to get to this point? Are there any definite choices you can make so you don't have to guess at the process? Yes! There are four steps that can be followed for most types of losses.

First, you need to *change your relationship with what you have lost*. Look back at what you've listed as your losses. Some are the lack of freedom from pain, the option to work, and the ability to sleep. You eventually need to come to the realization these no longer exist. They're no longer a reality. What helps is recognizing the change and developing new ways of relating to your condition. It's learning to exist *without* walking freely or working or being pain free. Memories, both positive and negative, will remain with you. Perhaps we can call this "acknowledging and understanding the loss." And you can do this with any loss.

The next step is to *develop your life to encompass and reflect the changes* that occurred because of your loss. This will depend somewhat on the losses and the extent of them. This may become a constant growing phase since changes and losses are ongoing.

The third step is *discovering and taking on new ways of existing and functioning* without what you lost. This involves creating a new identity but without totally forgetting who you were and what you had.

Finally, you *discover new avenues for the emotional investments* you once had in what you lost.[18]

Are You Stuck?

Getting stuck is a danger that accompanies loss and grief and other pains. The purpose for many emotions is to help you cope and give expression to what's occurring in your *heart* and mind. It's your way of reacting to the illness that has invaded your life. But instead of the trauma emotions staying around for a brief season, they remain for years. Emotions come and go, especially with chronic illness flare ups, changes, diagnosis, and everything that accompanies the hard place you're in. But when they seem like permanent residents, it's difficult to move on and develop an alternative lifestyle and new coping skills. One woman said:

> I am grieving. I've been grieving for some time. Why am I grieving? I'm grieving for myself, for all that I've lost. It's not just my health but also my daily routines, my hopes, and the future's opportunities that never will be. The control of my body and everything I might no longer be able to experience or do. But I'm really grieving over me—who I was and now am and who I'll never be.

To move forward involves overcoming denial and wishful thinking and facing the painful reality of your condition. You're going through major loss and need to deal with it head on. With chronic illness, loss and grief become constant companions, although the intensity will fluctuate. By now you've made a list of the effects of your losses. It's important to understand the impact this illness has had on your life. Many have said sharing their lists with family and friends led to greater understanding on their part as well.

It also helps to list expectations you have for yourself and your illness at this time. These may be realistic or unrealistic, but identifying them can bring a greater sense of reality and assist you in the grieving process.

What can you expect from grief?

- Your grief will take more time and energy than you ever imagined.

- Your grief will involve many changes.

- Your grief will show itself in all spheres of your life.

- Your grief will depend on how you perceive your chronic illness losses.

- You will grieve for what you have lost already and for what you have lost for the future.

- Your grief will entail mourning for the hope, dreams, and unfulfilled expectations you held.

- Your grief will involve a wide variety of feelings and reactions, more than just the general ones often depicted with grief, such as depression and sadness.

- Your losses will resurrect old issues, feelings, and unresolved conflicts from the past.

- You may experience a combination of anger and depression, such as irritability, frustration, annoyance, and intolerance.

- You will feel some anger and guilt—or at least manifestations of these emotions.

- You may experience "grief spasms"—acute upsurges of grief that occur without warning.

- You will have trouble thinking about memories, organizational tasks, intellectual processing, and making decisions, depending on your illness.

- You may feel like you're going crazy.

- You may find yourself acting socially in ways that are different from before.

- You may feel isolated.

- You may find yourself having a number of physical reactions other than your illness.

- Others will have unrealistic expectations about you and may respond inappropriately to you.[19]

- The uncertainty of what the future holds denies you the luxury of grieving fully.[20]

When you grieve, you're in the process of restructuring your life. Your world of beliefs is shortened, as well as having the order in your world disrupted. Your beliefs and awareness have been challenged, such as your vulnerability, safety, and continuous health or divine healing. Some of your beliefs may have been illusions. For instance, "There's always plenty of time to take care of that in the future."

Redefining Who You Are

This may sound strange, but you will need to relearn your world and reinvent yourself. The world you once knew and created around you has changed dramatically. You probably prefer your old world, but that's not a choice. If your efforts are directed toward recapturing your former life and lifestyle, you'll remain stuck and frustrated. You will never be your "old self" again. But you can build a new identity. You will need a new definition of yourself, including new roles.

What do you redefine? Where you fit in, how you relate to others, what you can and can't do, and what your daily life and routine will be. Remember, this is not a one-time learning experience. It's a process. You will also discover changes in your relationship with God and the teachings of Scripture. This can be a time of intense questioning as well as deeper confidence in Him. Actually this concept of redefining gives you hope. There *is* a future, although not the one you planned on.

Grieving is also about letting go, about saying goodbye. Too often people cling to what they know is gone or going, staying stuck in their grief. Many have found it helpful to write a "letting go" or "goodbye" letter to what they've lost, such as functions, vacations, social networks, people, specific abilities, dreams, trips, or the planned future.

With a chronic illness, there can be similarities to a sudden death in the family. In death a person is taken from you unexpectedly so you have unfinished issues. When this happens your mind is flooded with "I wish I had..." and "If only..." thoughts. You feel you were left dangling, with statements unsaid, issues unresolved, and no closure.

There is a condition described as "chronic sorrow" that involves feeling constant sadness with the ups and downs and ongoing losses. The chronically ill person often fluctuates from hope to hopelessness, and this makes it difficult to adjust to the new lifestyle.

You would probably have an easier time accepting your symptoms or pain or limitations if you were in your seventies or eighties. After all, isn't that when our bodies are supposed to deteriorate? But it's too early now! So you try to hang on to what you used to have and do. It's difficult to accept the reality and let go, but this is the way to redefining your life so you can get the most out of it again.

A letter such as the one following generates feelings, but it releases them as well. Writing a note like this will help move you along in the grief process.

> Dear Body of Mine,
>
> This is a strange letter. And I feel strange writing such a letter, but I need to. You were such a part of my life. I took you for granted, like so many things in my life. Who would have thought that the muscles in my legs were so important? But how else can I walk? I've tried to get you to come back, but no matter what I do you don't respond. You're still there, but you can't do what you used to. I used to be able to run, to jog, to swim a mile, but now I'm barely able to walk through the house. I don't like admitting it, but I need to learn to live without you as part of my life.
>
> I am now letting you go. I'm cutting you loose. I'm saying goodbye to the way you were and all you did for me. And I'm going to be thankful for what I have now. I don't like it but it's necessary. And when I start to dwell on the way you used to be and what you did for me, I'll say goodbye again and then look with appreciation at what I still have.

A woman with lupus said, "Grieving my losses served as a bridge, allowing me to celebrate my todays to the fullest instead of being imprisoned in my yesterdays and tomorrows. Grief was the key that unlocked the door to my adjustment."[21]

7

Your Fluctuating Emotions

an you imagine life without emotions? Perhaps there are days you wish they'd disappear, but overall they are a wonderful part of our creation. When Scripture says we are "fearfully and wonderfully made" it means our emotions as well (Psalm 139:14). They influence almost every aspect of our lives. God often speaks to us through our emotions, and they give color to our lives. They drive us forward, stop us completely, determine what we do and say, how we feel, and give voice to our inner voice. Emotions can give us strength or make us weak, bring us happiness or push us to the depths of despair. And they will control our lives unless we learn how to manage them and benefit from them.

Emotions are not just something you experience in your mind. You feel them in your body. There's a complex interplay between body and heart. The biological dimensions of your emotions are complex and a mystery. They can be one of the least reliable yet profoundly influential forces that guide your life. "Feeling" can be pleasurable, but it can also be painful so when there is too much negative going on, we often attempt to avoid emotions. But refusing to embrace them doesn't work for long and isn't healthy. Refusing to face the sorrows of life isn't what God calls you to in your journey. Jesus said, "In this world you will have trouble. But take heart! I have overcome the world" (John 16:33).

Your emotions open a door—the door to asking the important questions of life: Does what I'm experiencing make sense? Is there any purpose to this pain? Why, God? Listening to your emotions brings you back into the reality of living here and now. The psalmist calls us to face our experience: "Why are you cast down, O my soul, and why are you in turmoil?" (Psalm 43:5). This is often the cry of those with chronic illness.[1]

We asked a number of people with chronic illness to describe the various emotions they've experienced:

- "I have experienced emotions from 'just tired' to 'wanting to die.' I've felt depression and loneliness, hopelessness and misunderstood. Many, many emotions have been tied to this experience."

- "Bewilderment (before the diagnosis), resignation (about activities I can't do anymore), resolve (to find joy somewhere)."

- "Depression: It's rather depressing when I'm not feeling up to or can't do things I enjoy the most."

- "Anger: There are times when doing the required daily chores are overwhelming. For example, I get very angry with my spouse when he doesn't understand his help to vacuum the floor would mean more to me than all the presents in the world!"

- "Guilt: It's hard to 'just say no' to loved ones when they ask for help, so guilt creeps in when I don't feel like doing for others."

- "I experience extreme sadness when the pain is too great, and yet I feel blessed because I know some people that have this and can't get out of bed. There is sometimes a feeling of hopelessness, but I never choose to stay there. Frustration because I am limited as to what I can accomplish, and yet I feel blessed because I still have two arms and legs that work."

- "Depression is my number one problem. But I also feel alone sometimes, like nobody else can possibly understand what I'm going through. And occasionally I get angry. This really is *not* fair."

When you ignore your emotions, you postpone life. If you've not experienced many losses up to the onset of your illness, your journey may be even more difficult. The best use of the limited energy you have is facing your losses and grieving rather than trying to ignore them. Mourning will set you free to move on in life, whereas avoiding emotions is a self-imposed imprisonment. Grieving means *facing* and *releasing* your emotions. And it's all right—in fact, it's normal!—to feel what you're feeling.

Anger

It's all right to experience anger. Why wouldn't you be angry when you've received a painful illness you never requested? And not only do you experience raw anger, but many variations of it as well. Anger is feeling displeasure and irritation. In grief it's often felt as a protest, a desire to make someone pay, to declare the unfairness of what you're experiencing when you're frustrated, hurt, afraid, or feeling helpless. Sometimes the anger hits like a heat-seeking missile. There's no warning. No alarms sound. But there's a big and jarring bang. Another day your anger may be expressed in silent withdrawal. It's subtle, but it's there. Sometimes your anger is frozen. It's stuck or it turns against you.

Anger is all right as long as it doesn't get the best of you. Your feelings may be like the psalmist:

> How long, O LORD? Will you forget me forever?
> How long will you hide your face from me?
> How long must I wrestle with my thoughts
> and every day have sorrow in my heart?
> How long will my enemy triumph over me?
> Look on me and answer, O LORD my God.
> Give light to my eyes, or I will sleep in death
> (Psalm 13:1-3).

When your life has been interrupted by chronic illness, a normal response includes anger. You search for reasons or causes, but if none may be found your anger may be turned inward. Your emotion becomes judge, jury, and prosecutor. Often everyone in the family becomes angry. A spouse may become overloaded and impatient. Children may feel neglected. These feelings and subsequent experiences are normal with what you and your family are experiencing. Anger can consume much of your energy, and this is a problem because you may not have that much energy right now. Joni Eareckson Tada talks about emotions and anger:

Deep, passionate emotions force us to face questions we would rather ignore. For many of us, this is precisely why it is easier not to feel, to blanket our emotions with everything from distractions to drugs. But when we fail to feel, we are left barren and distant from God as well as others. We don't prefer hopelessness. Yet the alternative—anger—seems so destructive.

What do we do with our anger? Do we call it wrong? Turn from it? Squelch it?

No. We do much more. "Emotions are the language of the soul." They are the cry that gives the heart a voice. To understand our deepest passions and convictions, we must learn to listen to the cry of the soul.

> Long enough, God—
> you've ignored me long enough.
> I've looked at the back of your head
> long enough.
> Long enough I've carried this ton of trouble,
> lived with a stomach full of pain.
> Long enough my arrogant enemies
> have looked down their noses at me
> (Psalm 13:1-3 MSG).[2]

Anger is a strange and puzzling feeling, and it's not a signal to be ignored. It's like a special delivery letter with an important message. Anger is to our lives what a smoke detector is to a house or a dashboard warning light to a car. Anger is usually caused by fear, hurt, or frustration. And with chronic illness it could be all three. What is your anger trying to tell you? Someone once called anger "a servant bringing a message about our well being." But sometimes servants cause the house to collapse. Anger that goes unrecognized, unacknowledged, and untouched becomes an unruly and destructive resident that can affect the totality of your life. Anger seems to give some people a sense of control and power, but this can push others away—especially the ones you want and need to be a part of your life in a supportive way. Rampant anger hasn't been identified and dealt with in healthy ways, meaning it's been stuffed, repressed, suppressed, denied, or ignored. Joni describes this anger:

Anger has a dark side too. It has incredible potential to destroy. It digresses into a black energy that demands immediate release and relief. It despises being vulnerable and helpless. It relishes staying in control. It loathes dependence on God and so gains macabre pleasure in spreading the poison of mistrust. Ironically, this sort of anger—unrighteous anger—turns on us. It is a liar, offering us satisfaction, when in truth it guts us and leaves us empty.[3]

One of the indications of anger gone astray is blaming. It's normal to blame or try to blame someone else for our troubles. That's been part of our nature as individuals since creation and the fall of mankind. Some will be self-blame for what you're unable to do and how that may impact others. You feel unproductive and not worthwhile. And then you may blame family, friends, doctors, or the medical world. Blame will diminish when you begin to substitute the word "anger" in its place and then use your energy in a constructive way.[4]

Once anger gets a foothold in your life, it's one of the most difficult issues to handle so you can move on. One of the important steps is setting and working toward a goal of diverting energy in new, healthy directions. When you discover what you can accomplish and work toward that, your anger will diminish. Anger isn't the easiest emotion to control and channel, but it is possible.

Experiencing anger during the presence of a chronic illness is a positive sign! It indicates you're still fighting and haven't become emotionally numb and withdrawn from life. The energy of anger, though draining, can be used to motivate you to take action. Your background, life experiences, and church's teachings about anger may limit you in seeing the benefit of anger, but like our other emotions, it is God given. The best approach is to admit the presence of anger and use it, rather than letting it develop into resentment and bitterness. Consider the words of a woman with years of experience with chronic pain:

> I can now say, without a shadow of doubt, that when we get in touch with our anger and fully acknowledge it as our own, we find that it holds treasures that previously had been quite impossible. When we allow anger, we look beyond our perceptions and move forward to discover the preciousness of our lives.[5]

Identifying and facing anger's variations is an important step in the acceptance process. Use your answers to the following questions to learn more about you.

- I'm most angry at...

- I resent...

- I'm bitter at...

- I want to explode at...

- I want to vent my anger toward...

- What helps me with my anger is...

- I hate it when...

Each time we allow ourselves to feel and then appropriately express our anger, we are releasing negative energy and moving forward. The feelings we experience around our illness are not cast in concrete. Nor is there any great mystery about them. Each step we take to acknowledge and express them is one more step closer to letting go.[6] You might find it helpful to write out your anger thoughts and then read them aloud or share them with a close friend. You may also want to draw what you're feeling. The point is to express what's going on.

Guilt and Shame

Guilt and shame walk their way into the grief process. There are numerous sources for the guilt you may feel. The most immediate guilt comes from taking some responsibility for the loss, or perhaps the guilt is connected to a discussion that you feel contributed to the loss in some way. It could also be unfinished business you wish you had attended to, so you have regrets.

Guilt is unpredictable, and that in itself can create guilt. Some experience guilt because they're not recovering according to their timetable. This is where "should" and "if only" come into your mind. When a loss is unexpected or occurs sooner than anticipated, the tendency to blame rushes to the forefront. After you've blamed others, it's easy to transfer the blame to yourself. You say, "If only I had…" You imagine that if you had done something differently you could have prevented this. Do people really have that much power? If you had done something differently, could you have changed reality? Not likely. Or maybe there was something you always dreamed of doing but put off, and now you can never hope to accomplish it. You may feel guilt about many situations associated with your illness.

Doesn't it seem strange that you would feel guilt? Why be burdened by guilt over being sick? And yet it's as much a part of chronic illness as the pain and fatigue. It seems irrational and illogical. Why the shame? You didn't choose to get sick. Jean said:

> [Guilt is] the first response I have when I wake up. I try to discover why, but that doesn't work. I use logic and ask logical questions, but it's hard to get an answer. I finally talked with some other friends who struggle with invisible illness, and we have found something in common about our guilt—it makes our illness worse and feeds our depression as well. And the reasons for guilt seem to be the same: What am I doing wrong so that I can't get well? Should I have done this or not done that? Would it have helped if I had seen a doctor earlier or gone to a different one? The thoughts are endless and so is the guilt. If…if…if.

What can you do? Refuse to let emotional "guilt thoughts" take up *permanent* residence in your mind. There is no reason for these thoughts, nor should you allow space for them to exist. Yes, you may sometimes wonder if you're exaggerating your pain, but you're not. Your pain is real and probably more than most people realize. You don't have to deny it. When the Scripture talks about "taking every thought captive," these are some of the thoughts to capture, otherwise we end up locked in a mind prison. Every guilty thought needs to be drained from your mind. Challenge and dismiss them. How? By:

- writing down a guilty response or thought
- challenging it with "Where is the evidence?" There is none! "Where is the truth behind this thought?" There is none!

Write down those two statements that challenge your false beliefs. Keep them handy and every time guilt sneaks in, read them and take action. To help identify areas of false belief, complete the following sentences:

- If only…

- I regret that…

- I wish I had…

- I wish I hadn't…

- Maybe if I had…

- Maybe if I hadn't…

- I still feel guilty because…

- I feel guilty that…[7]

"If only" is a common phrase when struggling with illness. "If only I had…"

- not lived the way I did

- taken the medication sooner

- gone to the doctor sooner

- listened to the doctor's advice

- taken the trip when I wanted to

Fear

It's all right to experience fear. Fear is normal in light of what you're going through. And fears fluctuate and accumulate. They may come and go or you may feel a constant sense of dread. These are common responses when faced with the unknown and the unfamiliar. You may experience fear of being alone to the fear of the future, the fear of additional loss to the fear of desertion or abandonment.

You've lost control of your life, and that creates fear. What worked for you before isn't working now, and this too creates fear. The higher the expectations you have for yourself, the greater your feeling of loss of control; the more of a perfectionist you are, the greater your fear of loss of control and panic. Many fears are connected to the future. Fear isn't logical, and it's not predictable. And so you may be afraid of being consumed by fear.

Some people say, "I'm losing what I am." And that's true in many ways. Earlier we mentioned your identity is changing, and this creates confusion. The validation you received from how you were is changing or gone. Part of who you thought you were dies, so you end up grieving for yourself.

What do you fear?

> I fear...
>
> •
>
> •
>
> •
>
> •
>
> •

Because of the presence of your illness, you may be afraid. Do any of these statements feel familiar?

- I'm afraid of others withdrawing their love.
- I'm afraid of losing my purpose in life.
- I'm afraid of my illness getting worse and losing my abilities.
- I'm afraid of the pain and of it getting worse.
- I'm afraid of losing status, my job now, or the ability to work in the future.

- I'm afraid of losing my health insurance.
- I'm afraid of losing what I've worked so hard to attain.
- I'm afraid of looking foolish or looking sick.
- I'm afraid that I might die from this illness.
- I'm afraid of the future.
- I'm afraid of being abandoned emotionally and physically.[8]

Fear is a constant companion. "What's next?" is at the back of your mind. The fear of the unknown feeds your sense of helplessness. This is where knowledge is so important. Looking at your condition or illness squarely and saying, "I'm going to learn everything there is to know about you and then some" will override some of those fears. If you take on the role of a persistent medical researcher you'll be better for the experience.

Worry

Not only is fear present but worry weaves its way into your life as well. Whether you're experiencing grief or chronic pain, you may have a tendency to focus on the "What ifs." You worry about something and then ask yourself, "What if" and answer it with a disastrous outcome. Consider this:

> Worry comes from an Anglo-Saxon root meaning "to strangle" or "to choke." Worry is the uneasy, suffocating feeling we often experience in times of fear, trouble or problems. When we worry, we look pessimistically into the future and think of the worst possible outcomes to the situations of our lives.
>
> Worry is thinking turned into poisoned thoughts. Worry has been described as a small trickle of fear that meanders through the mind until it cuts a channel into which all other thoughts are drained.
>
> With worry there is a dread of something just over the horizon. When you worry you are preoccupied with something about yourself and in this case your illness.
>
> When you worry you don't handle stress or upset as well as

others. You're overly troubled by it. Worry has been called the fuel system for stress. When you worry, you add to your upset by coming up with several worst-case scenarios to your concern, but you're unable to know for sure which one is going to happen and this goes into your body.

Many Scripture verses describe the effects of fear, worry, and anxiety.

> I heard and my [whole inner self] trembled, my lips quivered at the sound. Rottenness enters into my bones and under me [down to my feet]; I tremble (Habakkuk 3:16 AMP, brackets in original).

> Anxiety in a man's heart weighs it down (Proverbs 12:25 AMP).

> A tranquil heart is life to the body (Proverbs 14:30 NASB).

> All the days of the desponding and afflicted are made evil [by anxious thoughts and forebodings], but he who has a glad heart has a continual feast [regardless of circumstances] (Proverbs 15:15 AMP, brackets in original).

Some with chronic illness have perfected the ability to use "what ifs." A medical doctor has a unique prescription known as a WIB or a "What if box." There are two ways to use a WIB. In your imagination you could create a "what if" box. And create it with a one-way slot going into the WIB, which closes once something is inserted and doesn't come out again. Whenever you create a "what if," immediately put it in the slot. Some have found it helpful to actually create a box, write out the worry on a 3 x 5 card and place it in the box.[9]

There is another simple way to tackle the "what ifs" of worry. Take every worrisome "what if" and turn it around to make it positive:

- "What if I never get over my worry?" changes to "What if I do overcome my worry?"
- "What if I forget to take my meds with me?" changes to "What if I remember to take them with me?"

- "What if I'm so sick I lose my job?" changes to "What if I am sick and keep my job?"

- "What if I never get off this medication?" changes to "What if I do get off my medication?"

- "What if those new people don't understand my situation?" changes to "What if the people really do understand?"

- "What if I'm too sick to go?" to "What if I'm well enough to go?"

Negative thinking creates more worry and anxiety; positive thinking creates anticipation, excitement, and hope. In his book *Free for the Taking*, missionary Joseph Cooke tells how he tried to suppress his emotions:

> Squelching our feelings never pays. In fact, it's rather like plugging up a steam vent in a boiler. When the steam is stopped in one place, it will come out somewhere else. Either that or the whole business will blow up in your face. And bottled-up feelings are just the same. If you bite down your anger, for example, it often comes out in another form that is more difficult to deal with. It changes into sullenness, self-pity, depression, or snide, cutting remarks...
>
> Not only may bottled-up emotions come out sideways in various unpleasant forms; they also may build up pressure until they simply have to burst, and when they do, someone is almost always bound to get hurt. I remember that for years of my life I worked to bring my emotions under control. Over and over again, as they cropped up, I would master them in my attempt to achieve what looked like a gracious...Christian spirit. Eventually I had nearly everybody fooled, even in a measure my own wife. But it was all a fake...The time came when the whole works blew up in my face, in an emotional breakdown. All the things that had been buried so long came out in the open. Frankly, there was no healing, no recovery, no building a new life for me until all those feelings were sorted out, and until I learned to know them for what they were, accept them, and find some way of expressing them honestly and nondestructively.[10]

There are two motivating forces in life: fear and hope. Interestingly, both of these motivators can produce the same result. Fear is a powerful *negative* drive. It compels you forward while inhibiting your progress at the same time. Fear is like a noose that slowly tightens around your neck if you move in the wrong direction. It restricts your abilities and thoughts and leads you toward panic reactions. Even when you're standing on the threshold of success, your most creative and inventive plans can be sabotaged by fear.

Letting Hope Drive You

Hope is a totally different motivating force—a *positive* drive. Hope expands your life and brings messages of possibility and change. It draws you away from the bad experiences of the past and toward better experiences in the future. The hope video in your mind continually replays scenarios of potential success. Hope causes you to say, "I can do it. I will succeed."

What can you do with your fears and worry? You can identify them and face them head on. You can look to Scripture for support. Psalm 37:1 begins, "Do not fret," and those words are repeated later. The dictionary defines "fret" as "to eat away, gnaw, gall, vex, worry, agitate, wear away." In addition to telling us not to fret, Psalm 37 gives us positive substitutes.

First, it says, "Trust (lean on, rely on, and be confident) in the Lord" (verse 3 AMP). Trust is a matter of not attempting to live an independent life or to cope with difficulties alone. It means going to a greater source for strength.

Second, verse 4 says, "Delight yourself also in the Lord" (AMP). To delight means to rejoice in God and what He has done for you, to let God supply the joy for your life.

Third, verse 5 says, "Commit your way to the Lord" (AMP). Commitment is a definite act of the will, and it involves releasing your worries and anxieties to the Lord.

And fourth, you are to "rest in the Lord; wait for Him" (verse 7 AMP). This means to submit in silence to what He ordains, and to be ready and expectant for what He is going to do in your life.

We encourage you to not let others determine for you what to do with your emotions or decide which ones are acceptable and which are not. You are the only expert on you.

Do you carry your fears around like a sack attached to you with a rope? In your mind, picture yourself dragging a sack called "fear." Okay, now see yourself turning around and cutting the rope with a knife. Reach out with both hands and take the sack. See yourself lifting these fears up over your head and then envision Jesus reaching down and taking the sack in his hands. Hear Him say, "Let me carry these fears for you."[11]

Now reach out to hope. Hope is the answer to the problems in your life. It's allowing God's Spirit to set you free from your fears and worry and draw you forward in your life.

Hope is not blind optimism; it's realistic optimism. A person of hope is always aware of the struggles and difficulties of life, but he (or she) lives beyond them and looks at the possibilities of tomorrow—even when today is not going well. A person of hope doesn't just long for what he's missing, but experiences what he has already received. A person of hope can say an emphatic *no* to fear and worry and an energetic *yes* to life.

You have several choices on what to do with your emotions. You can bury them or turn them against yourself. You can try to deny their existence and misuse what energy you have to stomp them down. You can vent them in a destructive manner onto those around you. But there is a better way! You can vent your emotions toward heaven so that everything you spew—bitterness and hatred and revenge and despair—never touches anyone else. This assault on heaven seems audacious and irreverent, perhaps even as inappropriate as desecrating the cross. Yet the Bible invites you to talk to God! The psalms, all 150 of them, provide a model for you. They show you how to express your emotions—not only positive ones, such as gladness and gratitude, but painful ones, such as anger and despair.

The psalms show you that when you approach God, you can freely speak the truth about yourself, about your circumstances, and especially about your feelings. God doesn't take offense. If anything, He invites such expression. He wants you to turn your emotions into prayers, however nasty they might be to your ears.

The psalms invite you to channel your emotions toward God so that in the end your emotions enrich your relationship with God.[12]

8

Depression

Chronic illness is a resident in your life that brings along another resident—depression. The beliefs we have about depression will affect our response to it. The sentiments written here could be echoed again and again:

"I try to do what I need to be doing, but I'm immobilized. The days are gloomy, no matter how bright. The nights seem endless. Apathy blankets me like a shroud. I eat because I have to, but there is no appetite or taste. I feel as though a massive weight is on my shoulders, and fatigue is my constant companion. I pray, I shop, I plead to lift the gloom, but it remains. I've withdrawn from everyone—from family, friends, and even God. Who would want to be around me? I know I wouldn't."

This is the painful cry of a person in the throes of gripping depression. For some it's an occasional heavy bout; for others it's a low-grade, constant depression. The message of depression is "You're defeated. There's nothing you can do. There's no way out. Life is hopeless." You probably already know what it's like to be depressed. Many do—major depression afflicts more than 15 million people a year.

Depression is a feeling of overall gloom, despair, sadness, and apathy. It's a move toward deadness, and hopelessness is the prevailing feeling. Depression is not like the sense of sadness caused by disappointment or loss. In a short while this type of feeling lifts, and even when it's your companion you still function relatively well. Depression lasts longer and is more intense. It can linger with immobilizing intensity, causing you to lose perspective and making you less able to carry on life activities. Depression slams down the window of hope, and sometimes it even draws down a dark shade.

Think of the literal meaning of the word "depression:" to move something from a higher position to a lower level. Frequently a depressed person, when asked how he is feeling, will say, "Really down."

Depression has been called the "black dog" of the night that robs you of joy, "the unquiet mind that keeps you awake."[1] The loss of perspective that accompanies depression colors the way you experience your life, your tasks, and your family. As one person said:

> "There's a real difference between being unhappy and being depressed. When I'm depressed it hurts all over; it's almost something physical. I can't go to sleep at night, and I can't sleep through the night. Even though there are still times when I'm in pretty good spirits, the mood comes over me nearly every day. It colors the way I look at everything. If my wife and I have a fight, our marriage seems hopeless. If I have a problem at work that I would normally deal with promptly and appropriately, I feel as though I'm a poor teacher. I battle with the problem of self-confidence instead of dealing with the issues in front of me."

When depressed you experience changes in physical activities—eating, sleeping, sex. If a lessening of sexual interest occurs, depression may be the cause. Some people lose interest in food, while others gorge themselves. Some sleep constantly; others can't sleep at all. Whatever the particular effects, depression interferes with your ability to function. And if you function at only 70 percent of your capacity, what does that do? It creates even more depression.

Your self-image tends to plummet. You feel less and less confident. You question your worth. You withdraw from others because of a fear of being rejected. Unfortunately, when you're depressed your behavior can bring on rejection by others. You cancel favorite activities, fail to return phone calls, and seek ways to avoid talking with or seeing others. This could be because of depression or your chronic illness. Not only do you want to avoid people, but you also desire to escape from problems...and even from life itself. Thoughts of leaving home or running away, suicidal thoughts and wishes—all these arise because of your feelings that life is hopeless and worthless.

You brood about the past, you become overly introspective, and you're preoccupied with recurring negative thoughts. Your mind replays the same images again and again. You fixate on the real and perceived wrong things you've done or experienced.

When depressed, you're oversensitive to what others say and do. You may misinterpret actions, and your perceptions can make you irritable and cause you to cry easily. You might exaggerate or minimize your own condition. Jeremiah, one of God's prophets, said, "Desperate is my wound. My grief is great. My sickness is incurable, but I must bear it" (Jeremiah 10:19 TLB).

You have difficulty handling most of your feelings, especially anger. Often this anger is directed outward, against others. But it can also be directed toward you, and this can feed the depression. You feel worthless and don't know how to deal with the situation.

Guilt is usually present too. The basis for it may be real or imagined. Frequently guilt feelings arise because you assume you're in the wrong or that your depression is responsible for making other people miserable. And often depression leads to a state of dependence upon other people. This reinforces your feelings of helplessness; then you may become angry at your sense of helplessness. You may feel this way already because of your chronic illness and now everything is intensified.

The hallmark of depression is the tendency to despair. It's common to feel worthless, useless, and possibly hopeless about life. Everything looks black. It's even hard to feel anything. It affects your ability to concentrate or think clearly. You may get through the day but not without effort, which is difficult since you feel fatigued. And the sense of worthlessness becomes so ingrained that support from others falls on deaf ears.

Depression distorts your perception of the world. It's like a set of camera filters that focuses on the darkest portions of life and takes away the warmth, action, and joy from a scene. A photographer is aware of the distortion created by switching lenses. The depressed person, however, is not keenly aware of the distortion he or she is creating as the lenses are switched. When you're depressed, you are partially blind without know-ing it. And the more intense your depression, the greater the distortion.[2] Even your chronic illness is magnified.

What do people usually distort? Life itself. Living loses its excitement and purpose. The image of God is skewed. You might see Him as far away and uncaring, separated from you by a tremendous gulf or wall. And how you view you is distorted. Your value and abilities have seemingly vanished. And intertwined within this is your chronic illness.[3]

Depression is built into the human system. In many cases, it is a normal and healthy response to overwhelming, challenging situations, such as chronic illness. But it can also be uncomfortable and frightening. Depression has been described as a cauldron of dark feelings. The best way to deal with those feelings is to acknowledge them.

Depression tags along with most chronic illnesses. Who wouldn't be depressed when struggling with a chronic illness, the medical system, and people's lack of understanding and care? There's a tension within most people who have chronic illnesses. You need to be sharp and alert to deal effectively with doctors and make crucial life decisions, but it's difficult to do this when your body isn't functioning that well.

If you're depressed, remember this is the most common symptom connected with chronic illness. You're not the only one going through this. In the Scriptures are many people who experienced despair and depression. Listen to the words of David: "How long must I wrestle with my thoughts and every day have sorrow in my heart?" (Psalm 13:2). Job, Elijah, and even Jesus (in the garden of Gethsemane) suffered.

> And taking with Him Peter and the two sons of Zebedee, [Jesus] began to show grief and distress of mind and was deeply depressed. Then He said to them, My soul is very sad and deeply grieved, so that I am almost dying of sorrow. Stay here and keep awake and keep watch with me (Matthew 26:37-38 AMP).

Depression is the second most common cause of disability worldwide, and it's expected to become number one in the next ten years.[4]

Perhaps you've never considered the fact that being depressed is a normal response in life. It is *not* wrong to be depressed; it's normal. It's not a sin to be depressed; it's normal. It's not abnormal to be depressed;

it's normal. There is so much that most of us don't know or understand about depression, so we tend to avoid acknowledging its presence because of stigma. But in a sense, we should embrace its presence. It's not to be feared but listened to. If it's present, there's a reason. Depression isn't a sign you've failed, but it is a message to you. Even when depression seems to come out of nowhere, it starts with a part of you signaling that something is not quite right. At the very least, it's a way of getting you to stop and think about your life—and possibly make some changes. It's all part of human existence and God's alert system for your body, mind, emotions, and relationships.

Why not pause and answer the question, "What is my depression telling me?"[5]

A physician from Johns Hopkins School of Medicine said:

> Pain and depression very often go together and depression is brought on by "real" pain, not imagined pain. Moreover, depression is often missed and not adequately treated, which makes it very hard to reactivate or mobilize patients who are debilitated by pain and restore them to normal levels of energy or vitality.[6]

The Roots of Depression

Depression comes in a variety of packages. In other words, there are numerous causes including family history. More and more research is being done on the question of whether depression or a predisposition toward depression can be inherited. "Inherited depression" has been defined as "sad or bad feelings that occur when biological, genetic, cultural, or psychological depressions exist in a family and are passed down to the next generation as an increased vulnerability to both healthy and unhealthy depression." Sometimes this tendency is disguised so well that it is hard to discern. The factors that are the most difficult to identify as depression are biological or genetic or both. It is estimated that as many as a third of those with depression experience it because of genetics. The more family members who have been depressed, the greater the possibility depression will be part of your life.

Depression symptoms may come out as addiction, eating disorders, or psychosomatic disorders. The tendency to depression can also be passed down by example, since people learn by observation. Relatives can pass down depressive ways of thinking and behaving.[7]

Who in your family tree was depressed? Among the relatives, who were depressed? You might find it very helpful to research this. You can begin by making a list of all your family-of-origin members, beginning with your great-grandparents. Include your aunts and uncles too. You may have to interview family members or close family friends, but it will be worth the time and effort. As best you can, rate each of the family members you have listed on a scale of 1 to 10 for their level of depression. Use 1 for no depression or minimal depression, 2 to 5 for increasing degrees of depression, and 6 to 10 for intense degrees of depression.[8]

When you think of depression, consider it in two ways. It could be either situation based or biology based. Situational depression is also called reactive depression. With all the losses we experience in chronic illness, depression is expected. Reactive depressions relate to physical, emotional, mental, spiritual, or relational issues.

With chronic illness, depression, no matter what the cause, can make your pain and fatigue worse, which contributes to the depression and pain, and the pain intensifies depression and fatigue. And all three impact your sleep. You're in a vicious cycle. You go around and around and around. Chronic illness has all the necessary ingredients to start a reactive depression. Does this sound or seem familiar to you?

But what about depression being biologically based? Depression can be caused by a chemical imbalance in your brain. Biologically based depression, including those caused by genetics, hormones, or disease, is the result of changes in your brain's chemistry. This occurs more frequently than most people realize. There is no doubt that the brain plays a central role in the quality of life and how a person feels. The following fatigue-inducing conditions are caused by a brain chemical dysfunction of some sort:

- addiction
- bipolar illness
- chronic pain
- depression/anxiety

- sleep apnea

- stress

The number one disability worldwide is depression. The number one symptom of depression is fatigue. Depression isn't always feeling based. It can be from a biochemical process. Keep this possibility in mind if you tend to berate yourself for being depressed. Here are the classic signs or symptoms of depression, using the famous acronym SADAFACES.

Symptoms of Depression

Sleep—insomnia

Appetite—increases or decreases

Dysthymia—(bad mood)

Anhedonia—(lack of pleasure)

Fatigue

Agitation

Concentration problems

Esteem—low self-[esteem] or guilt

Suicidal thoughts[9]

Looking more at the cause of depression than its severity, we can place it in one of two categories: biologically based or psychologically/socially based. Biologically based depressions, including those caused by genetics, hormones, or disease, are essentially the result of changes in brain chemistry. In general, they respond well to medications. Psychologically or socially based depressions, on the other hand, relate to emotional, mental, spiritual, or relational issues. Since there's nothing wrong with brain chemistry in these depressions, antidepressants play a minimal role in treating these. Psychotherapy is the preferred modality.

Biologically based depressions are sometimes called "endogenous depressions," meaning they originate "from within" your body. Psychologically/socially based depressions are called "exogenous" or "reactive" depressions because they originate "from without." They are a response to life's circumstances, such as bereavement, loss, disappointment, and stress. No matter what the type of depression, however, once it sets in, it impacts all areas of life.[10]

Your Depression May Be a Chemical Imbalance

For many years, those living with depression were blamed for their "weakness" and experienced prejudice. This was partly because depression was so misunderstood. Scientific research during the past few decades has firmly established that depression is a medical illness and not a sign of personal weakness or an illness that can be willed or wished away.[11]

There are genes that create chemicals within the brain that relate to depression.[12] If you could look into your brain, you would see several types of neurotransmitters, which are chemical messengers used to communicate with the system in the brain. There are four of these to be exact, which need to be there in proper amounts for us to be in balance. When one or more are low, a person is thrown out of balance and depression results.

Imagine you're baking a cake. You have all the ingredients in front of you, as well as the instructions. You've made this on numerous occasions, and it's turned out well. But today, for some reason, instead of putting in the proper amount of one of the essential ingredients, you only put in one third of what the recipe calls for. The cake isn't the same, and the difference is apparent.

Your brain has four essential neurotransmitters (ingredients). Let's consider what happens when each one is out of balance or low.

One ingredient is serotonin, and it's probably the most influential chemical we have. If this is too low, the result can be depression and anxiety, as well as a lack of self-control and sleeping difficulties. It's also a contributor to headaches, including migraines.

How can serotonin be replenished? Only your brain can make serotonin, which floats between billions of nerve cells. If you have enough, you function well. If you don't, you suffer. But some medications have been found that help bring back balance. Don't hesitate to discuss this possibility with your doctor if depression is a significant issue for you.

Another chemical is dopamine, which helps you stay sane. If this chemical goes out of balance, you might hear voices saying negative things to you. When you look around to see who's there, you're alone. You would also probably have difficulty hanging on to your thoughts. You might experience paranoia or become grandiose in your thoughts.

Can you imagine what it would be like if both serotonin and dopamine were low at the same time?

A third chemical is called GABA (gamma-aminobutyric acid). Years ago trains carried a person called the brakeman and, as the word implies, he had an important job. Can you imagine what would occur if he went to sleep on the job or wasn't there? The train would run wild. When GABA is low, we tend to do the same. This chemical assists in controlling our worries, helps with our shyness, helps with sleep, decreases physical pain, helps in muscle relaxation, and reduces drugs and alcohol cravings. It's also helpful in controlling mood swings.

The last chemical is norepinephrine which is the brain's version of adrenaline. If it's low you may experience sexual dysfunction, chronic fatigue, forgetfulness, lack of motivation, and depression. If the levels are too high you may experience anxiety, insomnia, and panic attacks.

Can you see why it's important to have these four chemicals in balance?

Some individuals have genetic factors that figure into their brain chemical levels. They inherited the tendency to have low serotonin, so they live their entire lives feeling sadder than others because of genetic depression. Their outlook on life is more pessimistic than others'.[13]

Dr. Paul Meier describes this problem:

> Without adequate serotonin in our brains, we cannot even experience love, joy, peace, patience, gentleness, meekness, humility, self-control—the fruit of the Spirit. People who inherit normal brain chemicals (80 percent of the population), and also practice the behaviors, thinking, and sharing of emotions and confessing of faults as instructed in the Bible, have joyful, meaningful lives with the fruit of the Spirit.
>
> People who inherit normal brain chemicals but disobey God's loving recommendations for us by becoming bitter, negative, controlling, secretive, dishonest, etc., will become serotonin-depleted and become clinically depressed.[14]

For years we've heard about the correlation between bottled up or repressed anger and depression. Now we understand more about this. Scripture has much to say about anger, including Ephesians 4:26-27: "Do not let the sun go down while you are still angry." If we have enough stored up anger, dealing with it draws serotonin out of the spaces between our brain cells, and thus other physical responses occur that we've already identified.[15] Eating the right amount of healthy foods with the proper amino acids, exercise, cognitive behavioral therapy, letting loose of anger, and learning to forgive are all part of the solution. Emotions and our thought lives are very much involved in modifying the chemistry in our brains.[16]

Our thoughts are often responsible for the onset or extent of depression. They can set off a plunge downward in our mood that can spiral out of control. Negative thoughts about a neutral or positive event can affect what happens. As one person said, "Our world is like a silent film on which we each write our own commentary."[17]

Unfortunately, we can't take these chemicals, such as serotonin, like a cracker and digest them so they go into the brain. Medications do help though. If you take medication for depression, never apologize for doing so. If we take drugs to regulate high blood pressure, heart problems, cholesterol, thyroid, and other physical problems, do we apologize for taking them? No, we don't. So why for depression? Remember, treatment for depression varies with the individual, so the medications and doses will also be different.

We need the benefits of neurotransmitters. They enable us to think clearly, perceive reality, and move. Serotonin is the one that allows us to survive. It influences a wide range of basic functions, from movement to moods. It works in conjunction with other neurotransmitters. Its function is like that of the conductor of an orchestra. It choreographs the output of the brain. When it isn't leading, there can be chaos.[18]

Perhaps you've been on a trip across country. You're on the interstate. The travel is going well since the roads are open with no delays. But then you grind to a halt. You're suddenly stuck in traffic. A mile ahead is a bridge, but there's a damaged section and you have to take a detour. You're now traveling at a crawl, which adds hours to your travel time.

Think of the interstate system as an interior map of your brain. A complicated, intersecting system of nerve cells connects your mind to your body. At the intersections in this nerve "highway," where an axon connects with other axons, there are overpasses: gaps where two cells almost touch with bridges (neurotransmitters) between them. Neurotransmitters provide the connections, the pathways, for electrical pulses (messages) to cross to the next axon.

In depression, these bridges become damaged, just as in the interstate illustration. The bridges are damaged because of a deficiency in a neurotransmitter made of such chemicals as serotonin.[19]

How can these bridges be repaired? With antidepressants. (For one of the best discussions of medications, and for additional help with depression, see Mark A. Sutton and Bruce Hennigan, *Conquering Depression* [Broadman & Holman, 2001]). Antidepressants go by many names, based on their chemical structure or activity and manufacturer. Some are specifically designed to help serotonin levels. Their purpose is to restore the normal chemistry in the brain. It's important to follow the guidelines of what was prescribed and use them long enough to be effective.[20]

Medications help, and so does counseling, especially cognitive behavior therapy. The combination of counseling with medication is effective for 70 to 80 percent of those depressed.[21] Eating healthy foods with amino acids is also important. Dr. Paul Meier suggests the three essential amino acids we need in our diets are tryptophan, phenylalanine, and tyrosine, as well as choline.[22] Following the principles of Scripture, including letting loose of anger and forgiving, make a huge life impact. Emotions and our thought lives are very much involved in modifying the chemistry in our brains, as we've noted. Exercise is also vital, but with chronic illness it may be a struggle just to get out of bed, let alone exercise.

Losses Tied into Depression

That loss can contribute to depression seems obvious. Whenever the awareness of your loss brings up an image of what your life would have been like had not the chronic illness losses occurred, depression may increase. Adjusting to chronic illness doesn't mean you like the changes you have to make to live. But you *do* need to acknowledge the changes you have to make. This is not a matter of giving up. It's facilitating your ability to discover new options.

One coping skill that is very helpful is to make your expectations realistic, says JoAnn LeMaistre. The most important aspect of this is the recognition that they are time-limited. Ask, "What can I do right now based on the way I feel at this moment?" If you have two minutes, what are you going to do? Check with yourself to find out what you want to do. Chronic illness or pain can often make you feel that you must surrender all your goals and dreams just to survive. But that isn't necessary. Instead, word your expectations this way: "Within the limits of my physical ability I will do whatever I want to do for as long as I can." Then define what you want and use every ounce of creativity you possess to figure out how you are going to make it happen. Creativity is *not* impaired by illness. When you define the problem, you figure out how many facets there are to achieving acceptable resolution, and then you put forth the amount of effort that is realistic.[23]

When you're sad, you may be yearning for whom or what you lost. Depression makes each day look as though dark clouds are here to stay. Apathy blankets you like a shroud, and withdrawal becomes a lifestyle. When depression hits, true and accurate perspective leaves. Depression can alter your relationships because you may become oversensitive to what others say and do. Jeremiah, one of God's prophets, displayed these feelings: "Desperate is my wound. My grief is great. My sickness is incurable, but I must bear it" (Jeremiah 10:19 TLB).

If you tended toward depression even before experiencing chronic illness, then your depression may be intensified at this time. Chronic illness is a never-ending crisis. Like grief, depression is a journey that feels like a passage through an arid desert. It's a long, exhausting trek through barren land. Just remember: Others have traveled this way. You are not alone in your sadness. Even Jesus was "a man of sorrows, and familiar with grief" (Isaiah 53:3). Nancy Guthrie, after the loss of two of her children, wrote:

> And so it is in our sadness that we discover a new aspect of God's character and reach a new understanding of Him that we could not have known without loss. He is acquainted with grief. He understands. He's not trying to rush us through our sadness. He's sad with us.[24]

A psalm can be a source of comfort, especially during those bleak lonely moments: "Why are you in despair, O my soul? And why have you become disturbed within me? Hope in God, for I shall again praise Him for the *help of His presence*" (Psalm 42:5 NASB).

God is present! There is never a moment that He isn't walking with you. In your illness and pain you may feel isolated, alone. And when you focus on that feeling, you forget that you are never, ever alone. It may help to say, "God, You say You are present. I don't feel Your presence right now. I feel Your absence. God, work in my mind so I remember that You are here with me. Help me feel Your presence and comfort."

As you draw closer and closer to your feelings of loss brought about by chronic illness and get more in touch with the perceptions of life that trigger them, share out loud what is occurring for you. To help you do this, complete the following sentences:[25]

- I mourn because…
- I feel sad because…
- I can't accept…
- I cry about…
- I wish…
- I can't believe that…
- I grieve for…

As you cope with depression daily or whenever it hits, these thoughts from the author of *Being Well When We're Ill* may reinforce your hope:

> We need to hear this assurance again and again. Depression is not a lapse in faith, so we can affirm these truths repeatedly:
>
> - God has not abandoned you. Though you do not feel His presence, He has promised to be with you always, and He has *never* broken His promises.
> - Your depression is not sin, but an illness. You do not need ever to feel guilty. For any past, actual sins that you have committed and for which you have repented, you do not need to feel guilty anymore. God has forgiven them!
> - You don't need to feel shame that you're unable to give thanks

to God or others. Shame is a symptom of your illness and not your fault.

- You are not worthless or hopeless. You are beloved of God and, by God's grace and healing mercies, this illness can be treated.

To receive treatment for depression is not a sign of your weakness, but of your wisdom.[26]

After David wrote, "How long, O LORD? Will you forget me forever? How long will you hide your face from me? How long must I wrestle with my thoughts and every day have sorrow in my heart? How long will my enemy triumph over me?" (Psalm 13:1-2), he said, "I trust in your unfailing love; my heart rejoices in your salvation. I will sing to the LORD, for he has been good to me" (Psalm 13:5-6).

There is your hope.

Recommended Reading

These resources will expand your understanding of depression and give you helpful advice for handling it.

Dawn, Marva. *Being Well When We're Ill*. Minneapolis: Augsburg Fortress, 2008.

Hall, Donald. *Breaking Through Depression*. Eugene, OR: Harvest House Publishers, 2009.

Sutton, Mark A., and Bruce Hennigan, M.D. *Conquering Depression*. Nashville: Broadman & Holman, 2001.

9

Suffering *and* Pain

S uffering." The very sound of the word brings a frown to the faces of those who hear its ring. Our typical response is avoidance: "I want nothing to do with that experience. Suffering isn't pleasant. It's not necessary. It's not what I want for my life." Unfortunately, the Bible says it's part of life either now or in the future.

Suffering is at the core of chronic illness. It is the human experience of pain, and the degree to which it affects the quality of our lives. For many, it's a constant. It never leaves. And it's what has now become "normal." And suffering is more than physical. It includes emotional and mental states. It ranges from very harsh to being like pebbles in our shoes that cause us to limp. Suffering changes our lives, our behaviors, and, all too often, our futures. It's one of the mysteries of life. God doesn't always explain why we go through it. And He doesn't have to, but that doesn't mean He doesn't care. Job persisted in asking God why, and God gave an answer to Job's long speeches. But He never explained the suffering. He just reminded Job of His power and greatness, which helped Job realize who he was as a human:

> Surely I spoke of things I did not understand,
>> things too wonderful for me to know...
> My ears had heard of you
>> but now my eyes have seen you.
> Therefore I despise myself
>> and repent in dust and ashes (Job 42:3-6).

Every one of us has probably prayed, pleaded, bargained, and even demanded that God heal us or at least make our suffering more bearable. We've cried out for relief. Some have received it, while others continue in pain for years...or for the rest of their lives. So when God doesn't respond by providing relief, what does that say about Him? And what does it mean to us?

Suffering seems pointless. Especially at first, it's difficult to say, "Yes, I can see why God allowed this illness to occur in my life." And even when we do get a glimpse of a purpose, we ask, "But wasn't there an easier way for me to learn this?" Suffering doesn't make sense to us. The psalmist cried,

> O LORD God Almighty, how long will your anger smolder against
> the prayers of your people? You have fed them with the bread
> of tears; you have made them drink tears by the bowlful. You
> have made us a source of contention to our neighbors, and our
> enemies mock us (Psalm 80:4-6).

Are there any answers that suffice when it comes to suffering? Will answers make you feel better? Answers are for the head. They often don't reach the problem where it hurts—in the gut and the heart. Joni Eareckson Tada and Steve Estes said, "We need to be reassured that the world, the universe, is not in nightmarish chaos, but orderly and stable. God must be at the center of all things. He must be in the center of our suffering. God, like a father, doesn't just give advice. He gives Himself."[1] Some Christians live by assumptions that are not necessarily biblically based. For example:

- Life is fair.

- I can control what happens to me, especially when it comes to illness.

- If I follow Christ and His teachings, no tragedy, such as chronic illness, will happen to me.

- If I'm suffering, it's because I've sinned.

- My body was meant to live forever and stay in good health... at least until age 80.

It is so important to deal with the assumptions and expectations of life before the realities of life confront us. When we don't, too often God gets the blame.

We know that God is all knowing and powerful. But did He choose you just to give you chronic illness and pain? Christian psychiatrist Dwight Carlson says,

> The belief that God is in control of the universe leads some people to conclude He has planned every last detail and wants every event to come about exactly as it does. Such a God would delight in pushing misfortune buttons; this God says, "Let's give Mary an 'A' on her English test today. Let's give Joanne a dent in her fender. I'll clog Pat's sink. Joe will get a heart attack, and I'll give Susan leukemia." Nothing could be further from the truth.[2]

And yet some believe this is what occurred.

> Many believe that we're special because of our relationship with [God] or because we've done something for Him, and therefore He will insulate us from the misfortunes of life. "It's time that God might intervene—at his sovereign choosing—but it is not our divine right to demand his intervention."[3]

Pain, death, tragedy, suffering—when they hit us we feel tormented, and age-old questions emerge: Why does God allow suffering? Where is He in my suffering? Does pain have any meaning? We're going to share a number of thoughts and ideas on suffering with you. You may disagree with some, agree with others, and become upset over some—and that's okay. All responses are all right. We ask that you consider what each person has to say and perhaps you'll gain more understanding on this difficult path you are walking. Delores Kuenning, in *Helping People Through Grief,* said:

> We all fear pain; yet from infancy it serves as a warning mechanism within our bodies to protect us from the hot stove or alert us to an inflammatory process within. But when it ravages our bodies, or the body of a loved one, it sears the soul and torments us physically, emotionally, and spiritually. *Why does God allow suffering?* we ask. *Does suffering have meaning?*

Daniel Simundson, in *Where Is God in My Suffering?* reminds us that "when we cry out to God in our times of suffering, we know that we will be heard by one who truly knows what we have gone through. It is a great comfort for a sufferer to know the presence of an understanding and compassionate God, who not only invites our very human prayers but also knows what it is like to be in so much pain. God hears. God understands. God suffers with us. This lament is heard by One who has been there." [4]

God is not uncaring. He walks with you in your suffering. Time and time again Scripture states God is good, and He cares for mankind. We also know that God is omnipotent. So what does His omnipotence mean to you? Sometimes we attribute incorrect meanings to "all powerful." Does it mean we're robots, and God causes every single thing that happens in the world? No. He is all-powerful, but everything that happens in the world isn't necessarily the way He wants it. At the creation of the world, He made people and gave us the ability and freedom to make choices. Because of our choices, and the existence of the devil, there are results now that aren't what God desires. He couldn't give us the freedom to love Him if we didn't also have the freedom to reject Him and His teachings. He wants us to love Him by choice. Consider this:

It is further possible that since God greatly desires individuals who willingly love, worship and follow Him, He had no alternative but to allow Satan to test them with pain, suffering, and misfortune. This is one of the major points taught in the Book of Job. Let me assure you that this does not mean God is not sovereign; in the Book of Job, Satan had to request permission to test Job, and God allowed it only within very fixed limits (Job 2:6).

Recognition of God's self-imposed limitations is the most difficult concept to grasp...Many ardent Christians will have difficulty with this viewpoint. But I am convinced that when God created the world, He set laws in motion which even He chooses to honor. The problem for us is that these laws intersect our lives in the most sensitive areas—in our suffering and misfortune.[5]

Chronic illness is one of those areas. What good can come out of this experience? A question that may have passed through your mind was also raised by the author of *When Bad Things Happen to Good People:*

> If God can't make my sickness go away, what good is He? Who needs Him? God does not want you to be sick or crippled. He didn't make you have this problem and He doesn't want you to go on having it, but He can't make it go away. That is something which is too hard even for God. What good is He, then?[6]

Your handling of life's losses will be directly determined by your understanding of God. So how does your theology affect or determine your response to your chronic illness? People usually put faith in formulas. We feel comfortable with predictability, regularity, and assurance. We want God to be this way also, and so we try to create Him in the image of what we want Him to be and what we want Him to do. But you and I can't predict what God will do. Paul reminds us of that: "Oh, what a wonderful God we have! How great are his wisdom and knowledge and riches! How impossible it is for us to understand his decisions and methods" (Romans 11:33 TLB).

God is not noncaring or busy elsewhere. He is neither insensitive nor punitive. He is supreme, sovereign, loving, and sensitive. We don't fully comprehend God. We too have unanswered questions about some events in our lives. But all of life's trials, problems, crises, and sufferings occur by divine permission. As Don Baker puts it:

> God allows us to suffer. This is maybe the only solution to the problem that we will ever receive. Nothing can touch the Christian without having first received the permission of God. If I do not accept that statement, then I really do not believe that God is sovereign—and if I do not believe in His sovereignty, then I am helpless before all the forces of heaven and hell.[7]

How do you respond to this thought? It can be difficult to believe. God allows suffering for His purposes and for His reasons. He gives permission. He lets suffering happen. He is the Controller of the universe. God is free to do as He desires...and He doesn't have to give us explanations or share His reasons. He doesn't owe us. He has already given us His Son and His Holy Spirit to strengthen and guide us. So even though we look at problems and losses and ask, "Why?" God isn't obligated to respond.

"Why?" is an age-old question. Job asked it again and again. Jesus asked it just before breathing His last breath on the cross: "My God, my God, why have you forsaken me?" (Mark 15:34). Yes, it's difficult to accept that God allows us to suffer. If you struggle with this issue, don't be hard on yourself. It's all right. We may not fully understand why or want to accept His choices, but God is God. Scripture does provide some reasons why pain occurs. Suffering...

> ... silences and refutes Satan (Job 1–2).
>
> ... gives God an opportunity to be glorified (John 11:4).
>
> ... can make us more like Christ (Philippians 3:10; Hebrews 2:10-11).
>
> ... can make us more appreciative (Romans 8:28).
>
> ... teaches us to depend on God (Exodus 14:11-14; Isaiah 40:28-31).
>
> ... enables us to exercise our faith (Job 23:10; Romans 8:24-25).
>
> ... teaches us patience (Romans 5:3; James 1:2-4).
>
> ... can make us sympathetic (2 Corinthians 1:3-6).
>
> ... can make and keep us humble (2 Corinthians 12:7-10).
>
> ... brings rewards (2 Timothy 2:12; 1 Peter 4:12-14).

When we find ourselves stuck in the gap between the way we think life ought to be and the way it really is, it's easy to doubt God's presence in our lives. He feels distant; we feel alone. And then we ask two basic questions of complaint:

> • "God, where are You?"
>
> • "God, if You love me, then why is this happening?"

We feel He is absent so we lament. And there is no need to feel guilty about questioning God. We ask Him because we believe in Him. Jesus said, "You will weep and lament, but the world will rejoice; and you will be sorrowful" (John 16:20 NKJV). Lamenting is an act of faith, an invitation asking God to do something. And God does answer! But it may not be in the way you expect or want. Michael Card, in his book *Sacred Sorrow,* wrote:

> Lament is the path that takes us to the place where we discover that there is no complete answer to pain and suffering, only Presence. The language of lament gives a meaningful form to our grief by providing a vocabulary for our suffering and then offering it to God as worship. Our questions and complaints will never find individual answers (even as Job's questions were never fully answered). The only Answer is the dangerous, disturbing, comforting Presence, which is the true answer to all our questions and hopes.[8]

Jesus responds to the pain we humans suffer: "Do not let your hearts be troubled. Trust in God; trust also in me" (John 14:1). I will not leave you as orphans [comfortless, desolate, bereaved, forlorn, helpless; I will come [back] to you]" (John 14:18 AMP, brackets in original).

Asking why is actually arguing with God. Job did this. He didn't walk away from God as some are apt to do. No, Job persisted in his attempts to understand what God was doing. Abraham and Moses also engaged in arguments with God. They didn't always get the answers they wanted, but they did continue to believe, and their strong and powerful relationships with God continued.

You want God to respond to you in some way about your suffering—especially at this painful time. But often He seems silent. This is what many experience. Our tendency in the midst of suffering is to search for some sort of meaning or spiritual significance in it. But if we were given a reason, would we really accept it and be satisfied? Really?

When you feel that God is silent, what can you do? Don't give up! Keep talking to Him and to other believers. Even if it's difficult to find meaning and strength in praying and reading Scripture, continue to do so. God is often silent when we prefer that He speak, and He interrupts us when we prefer that He stay silent. His ways are not our ways. To live with the sacred God of creation means that we worship a God who is often mysterious—too mysterious to fit our formulas for better living.

God is not our best friend, our secret lover, or our good-luck charm. He is God. The sacred can never be contained by our fervent prayers, or our theological boxes or our great need to have someone on our side. God will not be leashed. He will not speak on command.[9]

Strange as it may sound, we need unanswered prayer. Think of it as God's gift. It protects us from ourselves. If all our prayers were answered, we would abuse the power—that's the human way. We would use prayer to change the world to our liking, and soon chaos would reign. Like spoiled children with too many toys and too much money, we would grab for more and more. We would pray for victory at the expense of others; we would be intoxicated by the power we would wield. We would hurt other people and exalt ourselves.

Unanswered prayer protects us. It breaks us, deepens us, exposes us, and transforms us. Ironically, the unanswered prayers of the past, which so often leave us feeling hurt, abandoned, and disillusioned, serve as a refiner's fire that prepares us for the answered prayers in the future, *if* we are willing to look deep into the darkness of our souls and persist in prayer when there doesn't seem to be any reason to.[10]

Also remember the suffering of others, including God and His Son. Jesus' cry, "My God, my God, why have you forsaken me?" echoes the woes of many with chronic illness and pain. The appeal of Jesus was a desperate cry from one in excruciating pain. When you feel that others don't understand the depths of your pain, remember that a suffering and traumatized Jesus understands what you are going through. He suffers with you...and He suffered for you. The prophet Isaiah said of God's relationship to His people, "In all their distress he too was distressed" (Isaiah 63:9).[11]

If the cross was where God chose to reveal Himself most clearly, to perform His supreme saving act for humanity, then we have a God who suffers. If God chose to reveal Himself in a Man who was "familiar with suffering" (Isaiah 53:3), then we have a God who understands pain. In fact, suffering appears at the very heart of who and what God is.

God in Christ suffered on the cross, so we can't so readily accuse God of injustice when He allows us or our loved ones to be afflicted with pain. Dorothy Sayers wrote:

For whatever reason God chose to make man as he is—limited and suffering and subject to sorrows and death—He had the honesty and courage to take His own medicine. Whatever game He is playing with His creation, He has kept His own rules and played fair. He can exact nothing from man that He has not exacted from Himself. He has Himself gone through the whole of human experience, from the trivial irritations of family life and the cramping restrictions of hard work and lack of money to the worst horrors of pain and humiliation, defeat, despair and death. When He was a man, He played the man. He was born in poverty and died in disgrace and thought it well worthwhile.[12]

One person said, "Eventually we no longer ask, 'Why am I suffering?' but 'For what purpose can God's work be carried out in the midst of what I am going through?'" Reframing the question in this way makes you part of God's plan and saves you from self-pity. It helps you grow from a child to an adult—to become spiritually mature. Rather than feeling like a victim, you become a participant in life to help redeem what was lost. Asking "for what purpose" also saves you from the pain of the moment and gives you a future to embrace.

And when we learn to answer the "what," we can effectively "join...in suffering for the gospel, by the power of God, who has saved us and called us to a holy life—not because of anything we have done but because of his own purpose and grace" (2 Timothy 1:8-9). For in truth, "suffering ultimately calls *our* lives into question, not God's."[13]

What God allows us to experience is for our growth. God has arranged the seasons of nature to produce growth, and He arranges the experiences of the seasons of our lives for growth also. Some days bring sunshine and some bring storms. Both are necessary. He knows the amount of pressure we can handle. First Corinthians 10:13 tells us He will not let us be tempted beyond what we can bear. But He *does* let us be tempted, feel pain, and experience suffering. He doesn't always give us what we think we need or want, but He will produce growth.

In a counseling session with me (Norm), a woman shared her struggle. She'd been diagnosed with lupus and chronic fatigue syndrome several months prior and was upset because a friend had suggested she thank God for the illness she was experiencing. "I can't believe she'd say that!" the woman exclaimed. "That's ridiculous! It's insensitive. How can I thank God for this loss? It's disrupted my whole life." She continued to vent her frustration.

After a while I asked, "I wonder what your friend meant by her comment?"

"What do you mean?" she replied.

"Well, did she mean to thank God for this disease as though it were good in and itself or to thank God for using this so you would have an opportunity to change and grow and perhaps help others? Could that be it?"

"Well…I don't know," she ventured.

"I know it hurts, and you and your family wish it had never occurred," I said, "but it did. This can't be changed, and you feel out of control. Perhaps you can't change what happens in the future, but you can control your response to what occurs. This is something to think about."

She did think about it, and in time she came to the place of thanking God for being with her and allowing this time of growth. But she needed to come to this point in her own time.

"One day I thought about the choices I had," she said. "I could depend on God, thank Him, and allow Him to work through me. This didn't seem so bad when I considered the alternative."

Gerald Sittser knows what it is to suffer. His wife, daughter, and mother were killed in front of him: He confronts suffering:

> What about suffering? Does God's will include even that? I used to recoil from the idea, thinking it was unworthy of God, as if suffering and God's will were complete opposites, the spiritual equivalent of oil and water. I suppose on one level that they are. God does not cause suffering for the sake of suffering itself.
>
> In short, suffering has done me good, though I would never have chosen it. Not then, and probably not even now. I'm not sure that we should pray for suffering. Suffering just is, as unavoidable as birth and death. Sooner or later it visits everyone, no matter how rich and powerful that person happens to be. But I

do think that we should pray for the good effects that suffering can produce, all by God's grace.[14]

This attitude doesn't negate the pain of our illnesses. When we suffer we feel like the disciples adrift in that small boat during the storm on the Sea of Galilee. The waves throw us about, and just as we get our legs under us, we're hit from another direction. They struggled on the Sea of Galilee, and we struggle on the sea of life. All of us are afraid of capsizing. All we see are waves that seem to grow larger each moment. We're afraid. However, Jesus came to the disciples, and He comes to us today with the same message: "It is I; don't be afraid" (John 6:20).

We ask God, "Where are You?" but He is always with us! We ask Him, "When? When will You answer me?" We want Him to act according to our timetables, but the Scripture says, "Be still before the LORD and wait patiently for him" (Psalm 37:7). We become restless in waiting, and to block out the pain of waiting, we often plunge into frantic activity. This doesn't help, but resting before the Lord does:

> Often waiting is a time of darkening clouds. Our skies do not lighten. Instead, everything seems to become even more grim.
>
> Yet the darkening of our skies may forecast the dawn. It is in the gathering folds of deepening shadows that God's hidden work for us takes place. The present, no matter how painful, is of utmost importance.
>
> Somewhere, where our eyes cannot see and our ears are unable to hear, God is. And God is at work.[15]

We may not feel that God is doing anything to help us cope or get well. Why? Because we want recovery *now*. The instant solution philosophy of our society often invades our perspective of God. We complain about waiting a few weeks or days, but to God a day is as a thousand years and a thousand years is as an instant. God works in hidden ways. He's working even when we are totally frustrated by His apparent lack of response. We are merely unaware that He is active. Read the words of Isaiah for the people then and for us now:

> Since ancient times no one has heard, no ear has perceived, no

eye has seen any God besides you, who acts on behalf of those who wait for him. You come to the help of those who gladly do right, who remember your ways (Isaiah 64:4-5).

God has a reason for everything He does and a timetable for when He does it: "'For I know the plans I have for you,' declares the Lord, 'plans to prosper you and not to harm you, plans to give you hope and a future'" (Jeremiah 29:11). Give yourself permission not to know what, not to know how, and not to know when. Even though you feel adrift on the turbulent ocean, God is holding you and knows the direction of your drift. Giving yourself permission to wait will give you hope. It is all right for God to ask us to wait for weeks and months and even years. During that time, when we do not receive the answer and/or solution we think we need, He gives us His presence. Tell Him, "I trust in you, O Lord; I say, 'You are my God.' My times are in your hands" (Psalm 31:14-15).

I don't know if giving reasons for adversity or suffering helps or not. Explanations based on knowledge or facts don't always speak to the emotionally based question "Why?" "Adversity" is not a pleasant word. It's not a popular word. We don't seek adversity. We don't need to…because it will find us soon enough. It began in a garden. Adam and Eve started out with no adversity—no sickness or death or suffering. But something happened. They made some choices and life changed. Sin came in, and this brought suffering and death. This wasn't God's original plan or intention. Charles Stanley, in his book *How to Handle Adversity*, says:

> God never intended for man to experience the adversity and sorrow brought about by our forefather's sin. Death was not a part of God's original plan for man. Death is an interruption. It is God's enemy as well as man's. It is the opposite of all He desired to accomplish.
>
> Sickness and pain are certainly no friends of God. There was no sickness in the Garden of Eden. It was not a part of God's original plan for man. The ministry of Christ bears witness to this truth. Everywhere He went He healed the sick. God shares our disdain for disease. Sickness is an intruder. It had no place in God's world in the beginning; it will have no place in His world in the end.[16]

"Blessed is a man who perseveres under trial; for once he has been approved, he will receive the crown of life which the Lord has promised to those who love Him" (James 1:12 NASB). Not only does adversity lead to spiritual maturity in this life, it purchases for us a crown of life in the next. God understands the trauma of dealing with adversity. He hasn't overlooked the sacrifices we are forced to make when adversity comes our way. Therefore He has provided a special reward for those who persevere under trial. Once again we are faced with a conditional promise. This reward is reserved for those who willingly accepted Christ in their lives. These are the people who understood that God was up to something, that the adversity they faced was the means by which something good would come about in their lives.

Pain and suffering are related scripturally to endurance or perseverance. What does endurance mean in chronic illness? Perhaps it's the steady determination to keep going even when everything in you wants to slow down or even stop. To get through a long haul you need to have endurance. To endure means "to suffer patiently without yielding; to last; to continue in existence." Perseverance doesn't happen overnight. It is an ongoing process.

Are you persevering? Are you enduring? Or are you resisting? Are you mad at God for what He is doing? Friend, God wants to advance you through the use of adversity. He wants to grow you and mature you to the point that your character is a mirror image of Christ's. That is His goal for you. And adversity is the means by which He will accomplish part of this.

Why not pray, "Lord, I don't like this, but by faith I rejoice that You are up to something good in my life"? Eventually you will begin to see the "good." You will begin to experience peace. You will begin to advance through your adversity.[17]

Let's consider what Paul the apostle learned. He too said there is a purpose behind adversity: "Because of the surpassing greatness of the revelations, *for this reason*, to keep me from exalting myself, there was *given* me a thorn in the flesh" (2 Corinthians 12:7 NASB). Paul understood God was using the adversity of a problem in his life to further His purposes. Paul may have had a chronic illness.

In Paul's case it was so he wouldn't depend on himself and become proud. He was one who received an answer to his "why?" whereas you may not. Scripture does not tell us not to ask why. Paul saw something in his adversity that may be a struggle for some of us. He saw his constant irritation as a gift. Did he start out believing this? We don't know. We doubt it, but as he grew to understand what God was doing in his life he came to see it as a gift. His attitude changed. Perhaps he thought, *If this thorn in the flesh is going to protect me from pride, it is a gift from God. It can be used for some benefit.* I (Norm) have talked with some who see good things coming out of their chronic illnesses. I've talked with others who have discovered the other side of their illness. They don't discount or deny the pain and limiting efforts, but they see new character traits, new insights, spiritual growth, and opportunities for sharing in their lives. Some have told us they aren't aware of God's comfort at this time. Sometimes people don't look for it or give up. Charles Stanley said:

> We begin to doubt His wisdom, His goodness and at times His very existence. Doubt diminishes our ability to recognize the comforting Hand of God. It clouds our spiritual vision. Once we doubt God's goodness and faithfulness, we will miss His efforts to comfort us.[18]

We also discover from Scripture that during times of adversity God's grace is sufficient. He gives us what we need and don't have ourselves:

> Each time he said, "My grace is all you need. My power works best in weakness." So now I am glad to boast about my weaknesses, so that the power of Christ can work through me. That's why I take pleasure in my weaknesses, and in the insults, hardships, persecutions, and troubles that I suffer for Christ. For when I am weak, then I am strong. (2 Corinthians 12:9-10 NLT).

The Message Bible says:

> [Jesus said,] "My grace is enough; it's all you need. My strength comes into its own in your weakness." Once I heard that, I was glad to let it happen…Now I take limitations in stride, and with good cheer…I just let Christ take over! And so the weaker I get, the stronger I become (2 Corinthians 12:9-10).

There is a different way to view suffering and sorrow. God has a purpose in our suffering. Dan Allender and Tremper Longman say in their book *The Cry of the Soul:*

> He uses sorrow for the sake of redemption, all suffering invites us to struggle with God...what is this struggle about? It's our wondering why He's silent when we want to hear from Him, why we feel abandoned when we need His rescuing, why He seems harsh when we want His comfort. Perhaps you have felt this. The psalmist certainly did. He asked three questions.

- God why are you *silent?*

> Listen to my prayer, O God, do not ignore my plea;
> Hear me and answer me. My thoughts trouble me and
> I am distraught at the voice of the enemy, at the stares
> of the wicked; for they bring down suffering upon me
> and revile me in their anger (Psalm 55:1-3).

- God why have you *abandoned* me?

> Awake, O LORD! Why do you sleep? Rouse yourself! Do
> not reject us forever. Why do you hide your face and
> forget our misery and oppression? (Psalm 44:23-24).

- God, why are you *harsh?*

> You have rejected us, O God, and burst forth upon us;
> You have been angry—now restore us!
> You have shaken the land and torn it open;
> mend its fractures, for it is quaking.
> You have shown your people desperate times;
> you have given us wine that makes us stagger
> (Psalm 60:1-3).[19]

Our suffering has a purpose, just as it did for the psalmist. And it's simple: Suffering causes us to call on God. Our voices may be full of anger and complaints at first, but then we can move to praise: "I will praise God's name in song and glorify him with thanksgiving" (Psalm 69:30). In many of the psalms pain moves to joy. It is through the pain and suffering in life that we move to joy. Nowhere does the Scripture promise us a suffering-free life on earth. In fact, just the opposite. Look at the results:

> Now if we are children, then we are heirs—heirs of God and co-heirs with Christ, if indeed we share in his sufferings in order that we may also share in his glory (Roman 8:17).

> We have peace with God through our Lord Jesus Christ, through whom we have gained access by faith into this grace in which we now stand. And we rejoice in the hope of the glory of God. Not only so, but we also rejoice in our sufferings, because we know that suffering produces perseverance; perseverance, character; and character, hope. And hope does not disappoint us, because God has poured out his love into our hearts by the Holy Spirit, whom he has given us (Romans 5:1-5).

Suffering is a refining process for us all, but is that all? It may sound strange, but God can and will use our suffering to reach others. It's not what we want or would ever ask for, but it's the way God works. You and I have eternal life because of the suffering of someone else—of God's own Son. Through the intense and agonizing pain of another we have a relationship with God.

It's not that God can't reach out to heal you. He does have the ability and the power. It's not that He's unable to do so. Sometimes God doesn't respond in the way we expect or want Him to. And it's never because He doesn't love us. These are the messages made clear in the Scripture. God's love is abundant, totally unconditional, and His responses are based totally on love.

And suffering is not because we're unworthy either. God has never done anything for us on the basis of our worthiness...or denied us on the basis of our unworthiness. "Christ is the end of the law so that there may be righteousness for everyone who believes" (Romans 10:4). The reason for God's responses to us is simply His grace. And our lives can be different because of His grace. What does this mean?

> *Grace means there is nothing we can do to make God love us more. And grace means there is nothing we can do to make God love us less.*

Grace is totally free. It cannot be bought. It is undeserved, unearned, and cannot be repaid. Ephesians 2:4-5 says, "Because of his great love for us, God, who is rich in mercy, made us alive with Christ even when we were dead in transgressions—it is by grace you have been saved."

God doesn't say...

- "I love you *because*..."
- "I love you *since*..."
- "I will love you *if*..."
- "I will love you *when*..."
- "I will love you *after*..."
- "I will love you *provided*..."

Simply put, grace extends favor and kindness to one who doesn't deserve it and can never earn it. Sometimes our illnesses overwhelm us so much we forget the extent of God's love for us.[20]

We encourage you to consider all you've read in this chapter. In the midst of pain and exhaustion, think about how God might use what you are experiencing to touch others. He will surprise you. He is here. He hears you. He loves you.

Recommended Reading

To learn more on suffering, we recommend the following books. Some are written from a Christian perspective, while others are not.

Card, Michael. *A Sacred Sorrow*. Colorado Springs: NavPress, 2006.

Dawn, Marva. *Being Well When We're Ill*. Minneapolis: Augsburg Fortress, 2008.

Thomas, John C., and Gary Habermas. *What's Good About Feeling Bad?* Wheaton, IL: Tyndale House, 2008.

10

Rebuilding
Your Life

PART 1

When a fire rages through a community, when a hurricane or tornado devastates entire towns, when a person experiences a death or divorce, rebuilding occurs. And it also happens when your life is changed by chronic illness. How do you rebuild and get your life back the way it was? You don't. You rebuild and make modifications. Your new "home" may not be what you wanted or dreamed about, but you'll have a place to live and thrive instead of being defeated by your illness and living in a hovel of despair.

Let's look at several rebuilding materials you can use now and later to construct a fulfilling and satisfying life. Consider each one, and be open to new possibilities.

Attitude

People talk about it, encourage it, malign it, and still it confronts us often. "Attitude"—your attitudes toward life and illnesses—is a major factor if you have chronic illness and pain. Many are sick and tired of hearing people say, "Oh, it's just your attitude," or "If you'd just change your attitude you'd feel better," or "Get a positive attitude. After all, you're a Christian, aren't you?" No matter what your experience has been, attitude plays a major role. The Word of God even talks about it! "Consider it all joy, my brethren, when you encounter various trials, knowing that the testing of your faith produces endurance" (James 1:2-3 NASB). The word "consider" can mean "make up your mind to welcome or be glad about." It's basically an attitude you can choose.

But this choice isn't easy when you're *struggling* with *struggling*. What you used to enjoy, you don't enjoy anymore...but wish you could. And this dilemma can lead to even more pessimism, hopelessness, vulnerability, and depression. It's also true that the more negative you become, the more feeling helpless, blocking your emotions, and seeing the glass as half empty will impact your attitude.

Joy seems elusive when you're in pain. You think, "If my life were different and I didn't have this illness, joy would be possible." Tim Hansel went through this struggle with his relentless back pain:

> I was putting off joy until my circumstances improved. I discovered Nehemiah 8:10, "The joy of the LORD is *your strength.*" No truths are simple, especially those of Scripture. But as we pursue them and *participate* in them more fully, they begin to reveal to us a life deeper and more integrated than we ever could have known otherwise.
>
> My rage to live was real, but I had, without knowing or intending it, put a lid on it by saying to myself, "When I am strong, then I'll be joyful. When the pain eases, then I'll be joyful." I had enough excuses to last a lifetime.
>
> The problem was reality. The pain didn't subside. And I had placed myself in the position of waiting until things got better, waiting until I knew more of God, waiting until I had enough strength to be joyful.
>
> But through this profound and simple passage from Nehemiah 8:10, "The joy of the Lord is my strength," God reminded me again and again that I cannot choose to be strong, but I can choose to be joyful. And when I am willing to do that, strength will follow.
>
> The joy which I began to discover was radically different from the kind of joy (i.e., happiness) I'd known before. Above all else, this joy did *not* depend on circumstances. In fact, it was cited most frequently in Scripture as being in *spite* of circumstances.

Though the fig tree does not bud
and there are no grapes on the vines,
though the olive crops fail
and the fields produce no food,
though there are no sheep in the pen
and no cattle in the stalls,
yet I will rejoice in the LORD,
I will be joyful in God my Savior
The Sovereign LORD *is my strength;*
he makes my feet like the feet of deer,
he enables me to go on the heights
(Habakkuk 3:17-19).

I began to realize that it wasn't my imposed limitations that held me back as much as my *perception* of those limitations. It wasn't the pain that was thwarting me as much as it was my *attitude* toward the pain.

Joy is a process, a journey—often muffled, sometimes detoured; a mystery in which we participate, not a product we can grasp. It grows and regenerates as we have the courage to let go and trust the process. Growth and joy are inhibited when we say "if only," enhanced when we realize that failures and difficulties are not only a critical part of the process, but are our very opportunities to grow.[1]

Pain in life is inescapable, but misery is optional. We can't avoid pain, but joy is a choice. There are steps you can take to handle your situation. "I can't do it" or "I don't feel like it" can be an honest response, but there's another response as well: "In spite of… I will make the effort." If you can force yourself to behave in a way that is out of sync with the way you feel, your brain is faced with a dilemma: "What do I do?" Often the brain says, "Let's go with the behavior and give it a try!" This means instead of:

- "I don't feel like getting up" you say "I'm going to get up."
- "I don't have the energy to take a shower" is replaced with "I will take a shower."
- "I don't want to go shopping" is replaced with "I can and will go to the store."

- "I just can't make those phone calls" is replaced with "I can make two calls."

- "I have a feeling of desperation and always will have" changes to "I won't always have this feeling."

- "I am feeling vulnerable" changes to "I can feel stronger."

- "Pain is my life" changes to "My life is more than my pain."

- "My focus is on managing my pain" morphs to "I am managing my times of comfort."

You may be surprised by the results in your attitude and what you can accomplish.

Avoid Toxic People

We highly recommend you avoid spending time with negative, complaining, or pessimistic people. You don't need "basement" people around you; you need balcony people. Basement people live in the dark, damp, dingy cellars and drag others down with them. Balcony people listen to you, understand you, encourage you, and lift you up. They see the good.

What else can you do? We know we've said this before, but "Share your feelings!" Don't bury them. If you keep your feelings to yourself, the only person you talk to about them is you! And this reinforces their intensity. You want to drain them. Counter your excuses for not wanting to bother others by affirming that people care about you. Choose people who will listen and can handle what you have to say. Your immune system will thank you! If you're angry, say so. If you're frustrated, say so. If you're afraid, say so. It's all right. Be assertive. Be honest. Be direct. Don't apologize for your feelings. It's okay to complain a little, but don't get caught up in it. Remember there's a difference between sharing your feelings and griping and complaining. Going over the same situation and feelings again and again will only reinforce them. Be sure to let people you share with know if you want advice or just someone to listen and be a sounding board.

If you don't have anyone who will listen at this time (that's why support groups are beneficial), sit down with paper and pen and write out your feelings. Use as much detail as possible. Don't edit. Vent. Then read this out loud for you or as a prayer to God. This is what David did in his psalms.

Another interesting idea is to smile even if you don't feel like it. Sometimes the message from your smile gets to the brain and has an effect. One friend makes it a point to smile in front of a mirror for several minutes a day. She believes it positively affects her attitude. The nerves that are connected to these face muscles project impulses into parts of your brain that affect mood.

Along with smiling, compliment yourself. Often it's easier to praise others rather than you, but being positive about yourself will affect your attitude. If you do something well, give yourself credit. With chronic illness, the tendency is just the opposite, to look at what you used to be able to do and focus on what you can't do now:

- I'm not healthy, so I'm not lovable.
- I'm sick, so I'm defective.
- I'm of no value to anyone this way.
- People don't want to be around me.
- I used to have worth but now I don't.
- What type of a parent am I if I'm like this?
- If I tell others what I have, they'll reject me.

There is no positive purpose for holding a negative dialogue with yourself. So change your thought process! (This will take practice.) Look at what you can still do in spite of your condition and how you feel. Make a list of your positive qualities, characteristics, and abilities. Reflect on the value God sees in you. Tommy Walker, in his book *He Knows My Name*, describes how God views us. Why not read this out loud each day?

> [God] made me
>
> He planned me
>
> He knows me
>
> He forgives me
>
> He understands me

He comforts me

He listens to me

He "fathers" me

He wants me

He'll never leave me

He'll never forget me

He'll never give up on me

He cheers for me

He prepares a place for me[2]

Gradually build successes in your life. If it's unrealistic to clean your entire house in one day, clean one room or just clean a fourth of a room and save the other three-fourths for other days. Create situations where there will be positive outcomes. Do this enough, and you'll begin to see yourself as successful rather than mediocre or a failure. Don't compare what you do now with what you were once capable of doing. That's unfair to you. You're at a new place, so establish a new standard for yourself. And don't fret about what others may think. You can't really know what they think, and it doesn't matter anyway.

Be assertive in what you need from others. Let family, friends, and medical professionals know how to help you. Even when it seems doors are shut and no one is listening, continuing to knock is better than resignation—especially for your immune system.

Rebuild Your Thought Life

The most difficult conversations you have when you have a chronic illness are the conversations you have with yourself. Everyone talks to themselves. Some have positive conversations while others have negative. And when you're hurting it's so easy to slip into negatives. What you think feeds your emotions. Your emotional life has a direct line running to it from your thoughts. Many of your thoughts are automatic. They jump into your mind without any planning or conscious prompting. These may include visual images, a few words, or entire conversations. Often people slip into patterns of using "self-torture words" such as "must," "should," and "ought." When these words appear on the screen of your mind, they generate helplessness and frustratiion. When suffering from chronic pain, it's easy to create "the worst possible outcome" in your mind, which generates fear and depression. These thoughts, since they're automatic, are difficult to stop. It's hard to put a leash on them. One author said,

> Imagination is to the emotions what illustrations are to a text, what music is to a ballad. It is the ability to form mental pictures, to visualize irritating or fearful situations in concrete form. The feelings and the whole business builds up.[3]

Can you recall some negative thoughts you had? You may have thought they were realistic, but it's easy to move realistic thoughts to the negative side. Some people have found it helpful to write down their thoughts when their emotional pain intensifies. Often they're surprised by the connotations and connections. Let's consider some of the thoughts many experience in their struggles with pain:

- "I can't stand this pain anymore."

- "This is awful."

- "No one understands. No one really cares."

- "There's no hope for getting better."

- "I have to have pain relief now."

- "I can tell I'm nothing but a burden to my family."

- "No one at church wants to hear any more about my illness."

- "What did I do to bring this on?"

- "A year from now I won't even be able to walk. I can tell."

After reading this list, do you say, "Well, those statements are probably true"? Perhaps, but leaving them in a negative format won't bring any improvement. And it will affect your emotions. Now take each of the previous thoughts and rewrite them in a realistic format, such as: "This pain is bad, but I've handled it before."

-
-
-
-
-
-
-
-

The first step to restructuring your thinking is to identify your current pattern. Identify what you tend to say about your pain now. Don't worry if it sounds like complaining. And it's all right to experience and express any feelings you have. Once you've identified your thoughts, the next step is realizing as a believer the potential you have of restructuring your thinking. You're not helpless or hopeless.

Your thoughts can be changed! Remember, the One who knows your thoughts more than you know them yourself is your loving God. "All the ways of a man are pure in his own eyes, but the Lord weighs the spirits—(the thoughts and intents of the heart)" (Proverbs 16:2 AMP).

Even with your pain, you don't have to be dominated by a way of thinking that reinforces your hurt. You have been set free, according to Scripture. God hasn't given you a spirit of fear, but one of power, and of love, *and of a sound mind* (2 Timothy 1:7 NKJV). Soundness means that the new mind you have in Christ can do what it is supposed to do. Philippians 2:5 NKJV says: "Let this mind be in you which was also in Christ Jesus." This could read, "Reflect in your mind the mind of Christ Jesus." First Peter 1:13 says to gird up your minds. You are to change the focus of your thoughts from anything that's going to hurt your life. Fortunately, Scripture points you to the thoughts that will help: "Finally, brothers, whatever is true, whatever is noble, whatever is right, whatever is pure, whatever is lovely, whatever is admirable—if anything is excellent or praiseworthy—think about such things" (Philippians 4:8).

The next step is reframing your perspective. This means reworking your thoughts to bring balance, to make them more accurate and realistic. Let's return to a few of the negative thoughts we listed and consider some other possibilities.

- "I can't stand this pain anymore."

  "Yes, the pain is bad, but there are steps I can take to help."

- "There's no hope for getting better."

  "I don't know if it will get worse or better. It's done both before."

- "No one understands. No one really cares."

  "I'm going to look for the blessings in my life. I know there are some."

Most of us, whether or not we're ill, struggle with some of our thoughts. We all have this bent toward negative thinking, which is a carryover from the fall of mankind. And the ways in which we slip into the negative view are so common. We refer to these statements as toxic thoughts:

- *Black-and-white thinking* doesn't allow for exceptions or reinventions. It doesn't allow for good days or improvements. We use absolute words such as "all," "never," and "always." "Today is so bad I'll never improve." "There's no progress, and there never will be." "I'm always going to have these headaches."

  And then we tend to *generalize* about our lives. One negative experience or situation implies that everything else will be negative. "This doctor couldn't help me, so there are no doctors who are going to be able to figure this out." We create a *mental filter* that latches on to the negative or worst situations and ignores or discounts the positives or blessings. For instance, have you ever *jumped to conclusions*? You have a new pain or the pain is lasting longer than usual. Now you know it will last forever. And your life is over for sure. Yes, this isn't based on facts, but you just know you're right. Or perhaps your family didn't call, so you *know* they're avoiding you because of your illness.

It's also easy to *catastrophize* by imagining the worst. You begin asking the "What ifs?" and then go on to answer them in a negative way.

- Our illnesses impact our emotions so much it's easy to move into the world of *emotional reasoning.* We view and act on our feelings as facts. And since we live with discomfort, it's easy for negatives to gain footholds.

One of the constant steps in surviving a chronic illness is mental housekeeping. You will have some attitudes and beliefs that can help you for a while, but in time they will need to be discarded for better ones. Are your current beliefs helping or strengthening you? Or are they keeping you immobilized or stuck? Mental housekeeping is part of restoration, which can increase your quality of life. Illness generates the tendency toward negative thinking, and much of it comes out as blaming ourselves or others. Guilt may creep in because you think you're not doing "enough," or maybe "I brought on my condition," or "I'm creating more work for others."

It's important to develop an eviction notice for two words: "should" and "must." We've all learned these words too well. They are crippling, stagnating, guilt-producing, and reflect negative attitudes. Here are some phrases and their *balanced* counterparts:

- "I should go out and get that job done today."

  "I would really prefer feeling good today and go out, but I accept the fact that I don't feel well. I give myself permission to stay home and not feel guilty."

- "I must keep the house picture perfect."

  "Keeping this place spic and span is what I would prefer, but I am learning to accept what I can do and what I can't do."

• "My family and friends should be more supportive."

"It would be nice if others understood and accepted what I'm capable of doing, but I can accept where I'm at in my life. Someday they might understand more, but if not, that's all right."

Personalizing also creeps into your thinking. You say, "I'm not handling this illness very well" or "If I had taken better care of myself…" You make yourself responsible for your illness, for the lack of progress, for things you have no control over.

We encourage you to always look for alternative thoughts and words that give you hope. When you come across a phrase that uplifts you, write it on a chart. Keep the list handy and refer to it often during the difficult times.[4] Start using statements that begin with…

• "I can…"

• "I will…"

• "I will learn to…"

• "With God's strength and grace I can…"

• "I am…"

• "It's all right to…"

Now go back and finish the statement starters you just read. In fact, complete each one with three different-but-positive responses. You may be surprised by these positive phrases and how they will comfort and encourage you. You're not practicing denial. You're learning to be realistic, to cope, to live with hope, and to make a difference in your life.

Notice Every Positive

One of the struggles of chronic illness is the difficulty of being so overwhelmed by the pain and fatigue that sometimes the occasions when you're not in so much pain get overlooked. When this happens, you're missing out on a blessing! So when your discomfort lifts even just a little or for a short while, notice and revel in it. These times will also give you strength and hope during times when your discomfort is strong.

One way to accomplish this is writing a rainy-day letter, which is a reminder there are good days as well as bad. We've all heard that it's important to put aside some money for a rainy day or time of need. So why not write a rainy-day letter? When you have a good day, write yourself a letter about the day—what made it good, what you did, how you felt, who you talked to, your devotional time—everything that made the time special. Then put your letter aside. On days when you feel terrible and think you'll always be like this and nothing will ever change, take out the letter and read it. You'll be focusing on a positive memory and reminding yourself that there is hope for good days.

We all want to learn how to handle or how to cope with an illness that won't go away. It's easy to focus on the pain or what hasn't worked or what has gone wrong. Here is a series of questions to answer that may help you be more positive in your attitude.

- *"How have you been able to keep things from getting worse?"* For example, "How have you kept yourself from being even more depressed (or fearful or angry or down on yourself)?"

- *"How have you kept your attitude as good as it is?"* You may not believe your attitude is good, but it could always be worse. Give yourself the benefit of doubt in a positive way.

- *"What have you done to keep yourself from giving up?"* An example might be "My friends have been a support for me" or "My faith and prayer have made a difference in my life." When you identify what you've done, amplify each statement and give specifics so you can continue to do what has worked or helped before.

- *"What do you do at the present time to maintain your level of coping?"* Many people struggling with chronic illness fail to give themselves credit for what they've accomplished. Identifying what you've been able to do will encourage you to continue. The main principle is: Whatever you're doing that works, do more of it!

- *"What personal trait do you have that enables you to function on this level?"*

- *"What quality or trait do others say you have for coping with your chronic illness?"*[5]

These questions can lead to one of the most important steps in coping and moving forward—always focusing on what you *can* do. This puts you back in control, setting up hope instead of despair. Seeing the list of what you can do feeds your sense of accomplishment and optimism. You want to change your expectations and dreams and refashion them in relation to your current reality. Don't compare yourself to another person, whether that person has a chronic illness or not. Discover what *you can do* and give yourself credit. Ask, "What am I able to do now based on the way I feel and with what I have?" And after your discovery, thank God for this. And if you're having trouble identifying positives, ask Him to help you!

All chronic illness sufferers are looking for solutions to their illnesses. Unfortunately, many of these illnesses are lifelong companions, so the solution usually involves developing a different way of living and coping. And this starts with accepting where you are. With that in mind, let's consider what may seem like a strange question: "Let's suppose a miracle happened overnight and you were given the skills to make your response to your chronic illness better, which eventually resulted in a better quality of life for you. What do you think you would notice the next day and those following that would give you the idea that this miracle had actually happened?"[6]

Perhaps it was an increase in an ability, a decrease in symptoms, you had more energy to do things you wanted, or you gained more hope. If the quality of your life was better, who else in your life would notice, and what difference would the miracle make?

Is it hard for you to fathom such a question? Consider it anyway. For some the answer may be as simple as "I'd wake up and look forward to the day." What might happen to your response to your illness if you considered this each day?[7]

There are many suggestions for strengthening your body and your emotional life. I (Norm) have seen the positive results of one of these in the lives of others as well as in my own life when dealing with difficult situations, such as grief and heartache. It's the process of journaling or writing. It's important to write longhand because it helps the feelings and memories emerge. Be sure *not* to edit. Let your thoughts and feelings flow. You can write what you've experienced each day, your emotional responses to your illness and pain, and record your progress—large and small.

This activity will help you drain some of your negative emotions and strengthen how you feel about yourself. Writing can help you uncover lost feelings as well as identify the losses accompanying your illness. These need to be released and expressed. You have a choice as to the memories and experiences you write about. Some people just write about the negatives in their lives—the disappointments, the failures, the hurts, and the difficult times. This helps, but if this is all you focus on, it can feed depression. Some have found it helpful to take the next step and list the blessings they've received in their lives both prior to as well as during their illnesses.

Why not list several of your blessings right now and spend time thanking God for them?

11

Rebuilding
Your Life

PART 2

Y ou'll just have to learn to live with it." Too many have heard those
words from doctors, family, friends, and other relatives. Perhaps you
have too. Living with a chronic illness isn't easy. It's not like having
an intrusive boarder or roommate in your home. It has a bigger impact.
Chronic illness changes your meaning of life as well as your schedules and
future. You are forced to find ways to manage your life, handle the ongoing changes, and evaluate and often change the way you view yourself.

In your process of living a better lifestyle with chronic illness, there
will be a multitude of suggestions given to you by those who are on similar
journeys. Some may help and some may not. You may have heard some
of the strategies in this chapter, but consider them again. There are also
new ideas for you to contemplate and try.

One primary guideline is accepting the uncertainty in your illness.
This needs to be done before you can really move forward. It's a matter of
learning to live life without certainty, probability, and complete control.
You may need to work with an inexact diagnosis or perhaps none at all
for a while. If you give yourself permission to be in this state of uncertainty, you'll handle it better and move forward. After all, everyone is
really in this state whether sick or well. The difference is you're probably
more aware of it than most.

Another guideline is realizing that although you may not be able to control your illness, you can modify its impact on your life by letting go of unrealistic expectations. Letting go doesn't mean giving up. It just means you can't control your illness and many of your questions will have no definite answers. Some say, "I can move forward if only I get answers," but moving on isn't limited to receiving or not receiving answers.

A third guideline is knowing that even though you may lack total control of your illness, you do have control in some areas. One symptom that can be controlled to some extent is stress because much of it originates in your thoughts. If people say, "There's no hope" or "Nothing can be done," you can respond with, "Yes, there is. Christ is in my life so there is *always* hope. Perhaps I'll be this way physically, but I can still grow mentally, emotionally, and spiritually." Giving up self-blame, unrealistic hopes, and some expectations, coupled with discovering how God can enrich your life can give you more of a sense of control, thereby decreasing stress.

Finding the Right Health Partner and Approach

A great goal is finding the right healthcare "partner" to oversee and advise you on your care. It's vital that this person be in the medical community, understands the uniqueness of chronic illness, is knowledgeable and current with the latest information on your illness, and is open to alternative approaches. This person may take time and effort (and perhaps a little frustration) to find, but persevere.

You also want to be relentless in your search for information about your illness. Before choosing a new approach or the latest "cure," check it out with additional sources. Are the claims proven? Is the research accurate? Is the promoter respectable, legitimate, and knowledgeable? Are the benefits greater than the side effects? Be flexible and consider more than one approach to your illness and the way you live your life. Your values and perspectives may change. This can be a positive. Don't focus solely on what you've given up. Look for what's new—perhaps in ways you may not have considered.

A "cure" for your illness may not be found quickly or at all. Medical communities don't have all the answers. With chronic illnesses, finding a cure may not be a realistic goal for you. A great goal is discovering and deciding how to live the most rewarding life you can. This goes back to attitude and faith—and through these there is meaning to life.[1]

> Everyone responds to their illness in a different way. Chronic illness can be seen as an interruption. Some hold on to the belief that this is only temporary. It will be a struggle but the illness will be overcome. It's temporary and "I'll do what I need to do to recover."

> When you view your illness as an *interruption*, your focus is on recovery. You're willing to be in a "sick role" until your doctor cures you. Illness is seen as a timeout from the normal functions of life. It's a temporary halt and soon you'll be back to normal, is the belief. It's just a time to recoup. But as the illness unfolds into a chronic state a person may feel betrayed because all the efforts they've put forth has not brought about recovery. As the illness progresses they learn about the meaning of its effects and discover loss upon loss. It's a time of a lack of diagnosis, perhaps new diagnosis and then actual diagnosis. It's a time of prolonged crisis.[2]

Have you thought of your illness as an interruption? Or maybe you're like many who turn their illnesses into an *intrusive* situation, which forces them to accommodate it or else. Now it demands their constant attention. Now they expect symptoms and a constant state of illness that may never go away. Life is lived around the illness. The only thing in life that is predictable is having chronic illness. If this is you, your illness not only dominates your time, it's also dominating your life. It's always present and the focus of your energy. Its pressure is certain, and you live in uncertainty. Much of your energy is directed toward controlling your symptoms and trying to prevent them.

You evaluate your days in terms of "good" days and "bad" days based on how intrusive your illness is. How intense the pain, the amount of time devoted to it, the kinds of activities possible, how productive you can be, choices available or not available—all enter your evaluation of a day. If everything is minimal, it's a "good" day, but if everything is intensified and the illness is the center of attention it's a "bad" day.

Some people even *grade* their "bad" days. Many say, "I'm just not myself today." They've talked with friends and relatives and worked out arrangements that when this is said, nothing more needs to be shared. It's a signal to others to lower their expectations on that day and increase their patience. The one with chronic illness handles an intrusive "bad" day by revising downward personal expectations of himself and the day. And the criteria for good and bad can change. Some days are a mixture of the two.

Some chronic illness sufferers put their efforts into *containing* their illness. They attempt to not let it rule their lives. They want to appear as normal as possible. Can you relate? If so, a lot of your energy goes into keeping the illness hidden from others. It's not public in any way, you figure. You keep it under wraps and treat it as if it is controlled. If the illness flares up, this is just the exception. The illness and its symptoms are camouflaged. You want to look good and function well in public. If this can't happen, you don't go out. To cover up the illness, you learn to perform as though you're well. You find ways to hide the problem. If you're successful, you're fostering denial—that you're not really as sick as you thought and perhaps it will go away. When flare-ups occur—and they will—you blame yourself.

Chronic illness plunges you into a school to which you never applied for entrance. Who would choose such an experience? No one! Its courses include learning to accept help, honesty in communication, educating others, reshaping values and relationships, the way time is used, how to accept the changes and limitations, learning to trust, influencing the medical profession, growing in your faith and relationship with God.[3]

Or maybe you're *immersed* in your illness. Your total life is built on it. For many, regular employment is a thing of the past. Often the disease contributes to lack of sleep and difficulties in mental ability. It's all you can do to get through the day, let alone get to work and be effective there. When immersion in illness occurs, you face various types of dependency—physical, social, and economic. Your activity level shrinks, and the number of relationships you have tend to diminish. Every day seems the same. Time stagnates. You no longer share common interests with the people you know, and only the most long-lasting and significant relationships remain. Consequently, you turn inward and become consumed by your needs and feelings. Others are blocked out, including

God. Sometimes you aren't even aware you're walling yourself off. You start questioning who you are and ask:

- Who will I be?

- How will this condition affect my future?

- How can I continue to be myself while having a relentless chronic illness?

- What will being dependent do to me?[4]

To address those concerns, here are questions you may want to work through.

1. If I were to meet you today, how would you answer the question, "Who are you today?"

2. Who were you before your illness?

3. Who can you become?

4. What are the ways you have responded to your illness up to the present time?
   - unproductive
   - productive

5. Complete this sentence as many times as you can:
   - I used to…
   - I used to…
   - I used to…
   - I used to…
   - I used to…
   - I used to…
   - I used to…
   - I used to…

6. Complete this sentence as many times as you can:

- I can...
- I can...
- I can...
- I can...
- I can...
- I can...
- I can...
- I can...

Many people say, "Above all, I just want to get better. I'm not sure I'll ever get well, but I do want to get better than I am now." Perhaps we all want this for our lives. But we can't usually control getting better physically. We can get better at handling our chronic illnesses though. Some people's illnesses remain the same, some people do get better, some people learn to "put up with their illness," while others continue to deteriorate. So once again we come back to the issue of making peace with where you are and who you are. It's called *acceptance*.

In the case of chronic health disorders and medical challenges, the destination or goal is not necessarily to become well, but to learn to accept what life has handed you. It may not always be a welcome gift—this one of chronic symptoms and unpredictable days—but it can be an opportunity to learn more about your inner strength and the importance of faith and the people in your life. It is also a chance to use the gifts within that might have otherwise sat dormant. Sometimes learning to be compassionate with yourself is a far more difficult assignment than caring for others. Chronic physical pain or symptoms often force you to care for and about yourself in new and profound ways.[5]

Acceptance is the most positive and the most difficult response. Dr. Elizabeth Kubler-Ross said that acceptance means agreeing to one's status without struggling as well as without envy, sorrow, or anger.[6] Be aware that acceptance is not a constant state. It shifts and changes. Some people tolerate or reconcile themselves to being sick, but they do this for the immediate present and fail to consider what may be coming. They deny any conjecture of what the future may hold in store for them regarding their illness. True acceptance means, "I have this illness now and probably will the rest of my life. I will work on the present and know this will shape my future as well." Acceptance is living with it, and seeing the illness as part of your life.[7] Acceptance is embracing it and incorporating it, which means living with it rather than for it.

John Ortberg tells the story of a medical professor who came down with ALS (Lou Gehrig's Disease) in his mid-forties. He lost his ability to function in all of his limbs and eventually his ability to move or speak. He only had strength in one part of his body—his eyebrow muscles on one side. John wrote:

> And so for the next four years he used his eyebrow. With his eyebrow he could operate a computer. So with his eyebrow he could speak to his family, tell jokes to his friends, write papers, and review manuscripts. He carried on a medical consulting practice. He taught med students. He published a comprehensive textbook on endocrinology and received a prestigious award for his work. And he did all this when the only thing he could control was a single eyebrow. He said, "Sickness may challenge your body. But are you merely your legs? Your will is bigger than your legs. For your will is always under your control."[8]

When acceptance occurs, hope begins to grow.

Rebuild Your Hope

Hope is not blind optimism; it's *realistic optimism*. A person of hope is always aware of the struggles and difficulties of life but lives beyond them with a sense of potential and possibility. He is a possibility thinker.

A person of hope doesn't just live for the possibilities of tomorrow but sees the possibilities of today, even when it's not going well.

A person of hope doesn't just long for what he's missing in his life but experiences what he has already received.

A person of hope can say an emphatic *no* to stagnation and an energetic *yes* to life. Hope is allowing God's Spirit to set you free and draw you forward in your life. Listen to the story one man told me (Norm) after he chose to become a man of hope:

> For years I limped through life. Other people saw me as happy, successful, and satisfied. What a joke! My life was pain—just pain inside. And I was very clever at hiding it from my friends. I moved through life smiling on the outside and agonizing on the inside. I felt hopeless that my inner life would ever change. For years it did not change.
>
> But now I can tell you that a person doesn't have to go through life with crippling hurts and frustrations controlling his life. I made the choice to change, and my life did begin to change, gradually at first. But now I am free to live as God wants me to live.

This man laid hold of the hope we have in Christ and through Him found freedom from the problems and pain of his life. You may be feeling as he did at first—that you're stuck and that hope is an illusion. Wrong! Hope is a reality. It is available to help you choose and change and be blessed.

Have you heard people say that having hope is a matter of one's personality type? That some are born more hopeful than others? Is that really true? No! *Hope is a choice.* It is an option. Many things happen in life over which you have no control, but you do have control over how you respond to them. When you have hope, some of the pain of the circumstance is eased because you're looking beyond the situation to what will happen in the future. And even if the situation can't be changed, your response to it can change. You can choose to take charge rather than be victimized.

Hope isn't something you just generate by yourself. You can to a certain level, but *real hope* happens when your focus is on who God is and how He perceives you. Hope comes as you move ahead. When you take your eyes off Christ, your hope can erode, which can cause you to give up, fold, cave in, or live with resignation. Sometimes the erosion of hope is like an avalanche that is over in 20 seconds. A negative experience hits you hard, and your hope suddenly goes flat. At other times hope erodes so gradually you're not even aware of it. You go through life with no ambition and feel unblessed.

As a counselor, I (Norm) see hopeless-feeling people in my office every week. There are so many times when I wish I could reach out and give these people hope, but I can't. I can offer my optimism and positiveness to see them through temporarily. We can become so despondent and discouraged that we must rely on the hope of others to carry us along until our own hope returns or develops. If you've ever been depressed, you know what it feels like to have no hope. But hope can grow! Often it means not letting your situation or circumstances control you. When you are discouraged and hurt, God is still alive and sovereign. He still loves you, even if you don't feel His love.

The great danger of making your own plans is that they blind you to the presence of God. When Jesus the Healer passes by, you may not recognize Him as your Savior. "When Jesus saw him lying there and learned he had been in this condition for a long time, he asked to him, 'Do you want to get well?'" (John 5:6). Why would Jesus ask that? Of course the man wants to be healed! He's been trying for years. But there is a difference between being worried about brokenness and wanting to be well. What do we mean by that?

After a while people can get so used to the pain that it comes to be the most reliable companion in their lives. After a while they find so much meaning in suffering that to be made well would confuse them. It would also require major life changes.

So Jesus' question persists: "Do you want to get well? Do you *really* want to get well?"

"'Sir,' the invalid replied, 'I have no one to help me into the pool when the water is stirred. While I am trying to get in, someone else goes down ahead of me'" (John 5:7).

Can't you just imagine that if Jesus didn't interrupt him, the man is about to suggest that Jesus form a committee to devise a more equitable numbering system to ensure that the invalids would all get turns? But Jesus interrupted and said, "'Get up! Pick up your mat and walk.' At once the man was cured; he picked up his mat and walked" (John 5:8-9). Notice that Jesus didn't help the man be first into the pool. He didn't get him married or divorced. He didn't get him a new job that paid better. He didn't set him up with friends. He didn't do anything that would distract the man from his brokenness. What Jesus did was heal.

Those of us who have bodies that hurt need to remember that Jesus' healing doesn't necessarily mean a return to physical health. There is healing for emotional and spiritual health. We have been invited to pray for physical healing, but it is not promised. There is a difference between physical health and healing.[9]

Hope is directly related to moving forward in your life. It's connected to the process of healing. How? It prepares the mind and body to endure suffering, while at the same time helps you look to the future for something better. Hope never gives up; it keeps your dreams alive. Hope says there are always possibilities, options, and alternatives. You hope for what you don't know for sure. Is hope denial? No, *it's defiance.* You know what denial is: "I'm not sick. They're wrong. They misdiagnosed me." Defiance says, "I do have a chronic illness, but it's not going to ruin my life! I will move on and learn to adjust. I will overcome and survive." Sometimes defiance means you choose a new doctor, a new treatment, and a new medication. In *Peace, Love and Healing,* author Bernie S. Siegel, M.D., writes,

> You have to know what to fight for and what to leave to God. Your rights and your individuality are things you owe it to yourself to fight for, by saying that you will not be a doormat, by insisting that your doctor treat you with respect, by making sure you get answers to your questions, by wearing your own clothes in the hospital, by participating in decisions that need to be made about your treatment. But there are other times when you must have faith and trust, when you must allow God to handle the burden so that you can be at peace. This combination of a fighting spirit and a spiritual faith is the best survival mechanism I know.[10]

Hope perseveres again and again. It stirs you to action. Hope is what you believe to be possible in spite of the opinions of others. Hope is the belief in having a worthwhile future in spite of what is occurring in your life. On our survey we asked "How do you maintain a hopeful, positive attitude?" Here are several responses from men and women:

- "God gave me a precious friend and mentor soon after I became a believer. A precious little Dutch and Swedish older Christian. My Inge died in 2006. Words can't express the positive influence she had in my life for over 30 years. I maintain a positive, hopeful attitude by attempting to do as she taught me early on...I spend time in the Word and prayer daily. I try to pray purposefully...set a time if necessary, when my mind or body won't distract, to work on an eternal mind-set. Change, pain, and suffering are inevitable this side of heaven. Something she said so often...'to live is Christ.' It's all about Him. And what can separate us from Him...nothing. In any and all things we are more than conquerors through Him."

- "Being able to work at home (I'd have lost any other job). My faith in God's sovereignty. My primary physician (who also has stage 5 Lyme disease)."

- "Prayer and spiritual reading—*lots*. Especially material on suffering and how God uses it in our lives. Making the most of the good days—staying away from everyone on the worst days. Sending the family away sometimes for a few days so they can be replenished."

- "The Lord gives me all the positive backing that I need. I constantly thank Him for my life, for giving me such loving parents. Every day I talk to Him about something, and through that, the devil can't touch me...he can try all he wants. But nothing will ever come between me and God and living and loving Him with all my heart. As I have gotten older, I understand I'm in control of my emotions and keeping up my faith because I know I'm not done suffering and there is much more pain to come. With God I can do anything and go through anything. Amen."

- "I have built my faith on a sure foundation, and when I feel tremendous pain, I do cry. But then I pick myself up and thank God that I can breathe. It is a choice to have a positive, hopeful attitude. I have met many people that are in despair, and they are Christians, but my God is not a God of despair but one of comfort, encouragement, uplifting hope, and a *life* giver."

- "I pray a lot! I know the Lord has my best interest at heart, and He will provide for me. I have to depend on Him. I spend time with friends and do not dwell on the negative. Each day I make a list and try to accomplish projects (laundry, Christmas cards, sewing, fixing dinner, watering the garden, taking my mom here and there). I am very much a type-A personality, and I need to feel like I've achieved goals each day. My friends say I have a great attitude—I hope so!"

What Can You Do Now?

1. *Take a hope inventory.* What gives you hope? What contributes to a feeling of hopelessness? Monitor your thoughts and feelings. Discover what you can do to bring hope to areas of your life where it's lacking.

2. *Find hope experts.* They're the people who know how to keep hope alive despite life's ups and downs.

3. *Appoint a hope committee.* The people in your life can make or break your hope. It's important to surround yourself with people who give you hope.

4. *Be prepared to deal with hope snatchers.* In every universe there are black holes. Just as you know hope experts, you also are acquainted with those who specialize in hopelessness. Avoid them as much as possible.

5. *Know where your hope is.* Figure out what in life brings you hope.

6. *Set a goal; get a purpose.* Whatever it is, make sure your goal keeps your attention and challenges you. If you don't have a purpose in life, get one.

7. *Be your own "thought police."* Make sure your mind obeys the laws of hope. If you catch yourself thinking hopeless thoughts, switch gears.

8. *Speak hope.* Like thoughts, words are powerful. Think and speak aloud hope.

9. *Hope in the past.* Make your memories real. Most of us can remember times in our lives when some situations looked hopeless and yet we survived. Remember how well hope has worked in the past.

10. *Hope in the future.* When you're struggling with serious illness or other difficulties, it's easy to become overwhelmed and forget the other, ongoing aspects of your life. Planning for the future is a way to defy hopelessness.[11]

We would like you to do something for two weeks. Although two weeks is just 14 days, this brief assignment can radically change your attitude and outlook. It's very simple. Read each of the following *aloud* every day for the next two weeks. Read them with feeling. Read them with emphasis. Grasp their meaning and significance. Reflect on your outlook and adjust them as needed. Experience the blessings that will come from these words.

- We have peace with God through our Lord Jesus Christ, through whom we have gained access by faith into this grace in which we now stand (Romans 5:1).

- For in this hope we were saved. But hope that is seen is no hope at all. Who hopes for what he already has? But if we hope for what we do not yet have, we wait for it patiently (Romans 8:24-25).

- May the God of hope fill you with all joy and peace as you trust in him, so that you may overflow with hope by the power of the Holy Spirit (Romans 15:13).

- And now these three things remain: faith, hope and love. But the greatest of these is love (1 Corinthians 13:13).

- By faith we eagerly await through the Spirit the righteousness for which we hope (Galatians 5:5).

- I pray also that the eyes of your heart may be enlightened in order that you may know the hope to which he has called you, the riches of his glorious inheritance in the saints (Ephesians 1:18).

- We have heard of your faith in Christ Jesus and of the love you have for all the saints—the faith and love that spring from the hope that is stored up for you in heaven and that you have already heard about in the word of truth, the gospel (Colossians 1:4-5).

- God has chosen to make known among the Gentiles the glorious riches of this mystery, which is Christ in you, the hope of glory (Colossians 1:27).

- Paul, an apostle of Christ Jesus by the command of God our Savior and of Christ Jesus our hope (1 Timothy 1:1).

- [The grace of God] teaches us to say "No" to ungodliness and worldly passions, and to live self-controlled, upright, and godly lives in this present age, while we wait for the blessed hope—the glorious appearing of our great God and Savior, Jesus Christ (Titus 2:12-13).

- We have this hope as an anchor for the soul, firm and secure. It enters the inner sanctuary behind the curtain, where Jesus, who went before us, has entered on our behalf (Hebrews 6:19-20).

- Prepare your minds for action; be self-controlled; set your hope fully on the grace to be given you when Jesus Christ is revealed (1 Peter 1:13).

Two weeks. You can do this for two weeks. Pray that God will write these truths on your heart, and then see what happens.

Recommended Reading

We encourage you to learn more by reading the following books. Some are written from a Christian perspective while others are not.

Dawn, Marva. *Being Well When We're Ill*. Minneapolis: Augsburg Fortress, 2008.

Hayford, Jack. *Hope for a Hopeless Day*. Ventura, CA: Regal Books, 2007.

12

Helping Others Help You

Your family and friends are greatly impacted by your chronic illness. As much as you didn't want your illness, neither did they. Just as abuse or substance use affects others, so does this illness you have. Just as you struggle with understanding it and what to do with your life, so do they. Added to their struggle is how to respond to you in a helpful, supportive way. This chapter is not so much for you, but for your family and friends. We suggest you personalize this chapter by adding your own suggestions and guidelines and then asking them to read it.

❦

If you know someone who has to deal with chronic illness or pain, this chapter is for you. Have you wondered how you can help? One area is helping your family member or friend deal with the emotional challenges. You have several options. You can retreat and eventually leave the relationship. You can fall into the trap of blaming yourself or the person with the illness for the changes in your relationship. (But blaming solves nothing and is a waste of energy.) You can refuse to adjust or help, meaning you and your family member or friend will experience frustration. Or you can adjust and respond in a positive and helpful way.

What to Avoid

Let's consider two roles or responses to avoid. One is that of hero or savior. This is someone who dives in to help the sufferer "get cured." This person rushes in to take care of everything, pulling the sufferer along. It's admirable that you want to save the person from his or her pain and misery, but you can't really do that. You'll soon experience disappointment and eventually give up.

Becoming a martyr is another easy response to fall into. Martyrs care for the ill person, but their focus is on themselves. "What did I ever do to deserve this?" goes through their minds. Or, "Now we can't just be spontaneous. This isn't fun anymore. There's too much work involved in doing things with you…but I'll do it." Often martyrs let others know about their plight.

Positive Steps for Both of You

One therapist suggested looking at yourself as a pioneer in a new land. The early pioneers sought out the unknown and built their lives. They rarely went alone, and usually shared the experience. They also paved the way for others.

You are more than a helper of someone with a chronic illness. And the person with chronic illness is more than the disease. Ask, "How would I respond to someone or view someone with a broken arm or leg? Would that change our relationship very much?" This approach helps you see your loved one in the same light even though the chronic illness could last a long time. Your life is going to change, and the more serious the illness, the greater the impact.

One thing that will really help is accepting the reality of your family member or friend's illness as soon as possible. This may involve coming to grips with your own disbelief or denial. Become as informed as possible about the illness, but let your loved one guide you in what resources to access and pursue. You'll encounter the temptation to search for resources that promise a cure and then insist your family member or friend follow up on what you've found. It's natural to want to be helpful and try to discover what might have been missed. Reading the rest of this book may help you better understand the world of someone with a chronic illness.

You will have a mixture of mental and emotional reactions to the illness as well as to the afflicted person. Work through your feelings. We know you want to help rather than add a burden to your loved one's already stressful and painful life.

Make sure you have others to support and help *you* as you are helping your loved one. Talk openly and freely with supportive people, and share your own fears and concerns. Your loved-one's chronic illness has a big impact on you too.

Work toward balance in your life. It's so easy to focus on the illness and other negatives when you're helping someone suffering. You need positive input and positive experiences. Beware of the tendency to neglect your own emotional and spiritual needs. Time away from the person suffering, no matter how brief, is important. Periodically ask yourself if you're getting sufficient sleep, food, and relief. And don't expect perfection from yourself. In caring for your loved one, you won't always know what to do or say. This is also a time when some of your own areas of weakness may seem to be accentuated. The ill person may not always be able to guide you in what he or she needs, so there could be a great deal of trial and error. Be patient with yourself.

Your family member or friend may need an advocate medically speaking, which means you may want to learn as much as you can about the medical system. You might be able to assist by making a list of questions and concerns so the suffering person can remember what to bring up at doctors' visits. In fact, he or she may ask you to go with them to take notes.

You will experience loss and grief at this time, and how much depends on the closeness between you and the one who is ill. If the person is a spouse, your life will be as disrupted as his or hers and will probably never be the same. Please don't try to handle the situation by yourself. Draw on the strength and wisdom of others.[1]

When you respond to the ill person, don't treat him or her as an invalid. What you say, how you say it, and even nonverbal gestures or expressions may imply you think the person is helpless. Don't do for the sick person anything he or she can do.

Your loved one doesn't need rescued—only assisted when and where necessary. Avoid plunging in and taking over and doing things for the person. Ask first, and if told your help isn't needed, step back. Avoid

saying, "You're not able to do that" or "This might be too much for you."
You're a helper, an assistant, not a caretaker.

Don't expect the person to feel better since most often they won't. This
is hard. Don't act disappointed that he or she isn't better. Be careful with
the look on your face or your words. An "Oh, you're not any better" can
reinforce your loved one's own disappointment and discouragement.

If the ill person isn't feeling well, let him or her explain if the person
wants to. Don't bombard the person with questions to try to drag out
the specifics. Your person isn't doing well because of the chronic illness.
This is what happens. The ill person may have "up" days or better days,
but don't assume each day will now be like this. An hour later the pain
may return with a vengeance. Don't be overly hopeful by saying maybe
the person has turned the corner and will experience better days from
now on. Avoid saying, "Oh, you look so much better" or "You sound
like you're better" with hope in your voice. Chronic illness symptoms
fluctuate a lot.

Your loved one has limitations you may be unaware of, so wait until
he or she lets you know how he or she is doing. Don't assume just because
he's up and doing housework that he'll be able to do this for another hour.
Avoid saying, "Remember how well you did yesterday? If you just set your
mind to it, you'll be able to do it again." "Setting your mind to it" has
nothing to do with chronic illness. Chronic illness is physical and real.

Don't suggest that by getting out and doing something your loved
one will feel better. The activity may make the situation worse by doing
it or worse because the person can't do it.

Abide by your loved one's schedule for eating, what he eats, and when
he needs to take his medicine. A simple comment like "You take a lot of
pills, don't you?" can be upsetting. A difficult thing to remember and
accept is that your loved one *is not* working toward getting well and then
rebuilding a life. Rather he or she is working on rebuilding and having a
life *while* enduring the chronic illness. Please accept this reality.

One of the worst things to do is to suggest cures. The ill person has
probably heard so many of these by now...and tried a number of them.
If you hear of one, investigate it thoroughly and don't become excited
because someone had a friend who was "cured" by "such and such." Everyone is looking for answers and cures.

Comments can hurt and be more insensitive than we realize. Some of the worst things to say are:

- "This must be God's will for your life."
- "You're going to grow spiritually through this."
- "You need to have more faith."
- "You need to pray more."
- "God never gives us more than we can handle."
- "I know people who are worse."
- "You've got to be strong for your kids."
- "Why not go back to work? It could help you."

What About You?

What can you expect in terms of your emotional reaction? At first it may be a mixture of shock and confusion and thinking you're going crazy. Another companion emotion will be some fear and anxiety about the current situation and the future. You may experience depression as your family member or friend's condition continues and seems endless. And then there's anger—at the illness, at how your life has changed, at the ill person, at yourself, at others who don't help you, at God, at the doctors, at the hospital. Guilt may work itself in by saying you're not doing enough or for getting angry at your loved one. Grief over your losses and the losses of the ill person will occur. All these emotions may accumulate as time goes on. The closer you are to this person, the more intense your feelings.

You may experience a fluctuation of feelings as you continue helping. Remember, the more exhausted you become, the more your emotions tend to intensify. Be careful not to overdo, and make sure you take care of you.

Do you find yourself becoming more frustrated or irritable? That's not uncommon. Even loneliness occurs because the more time you spend helping, the less time you have to spend with others. And you can't help but notice how others go on with their lives while yours may feel like it's at a standstill. If you're someone who needs to be in control, you may also feel a sense of futility and helplessness weighing upon you because you may be doing and saying the same things day after day. You may feel a sense of shame over your inability to help more or for some of your negative thoughts and feelings at this time.

If you don't express your emotions, they will accumulate and, at times, come out in ways you may not want. You need someone or some way to vent your feelings, whether it's to a friend, in a support group, or by journaling. It's better to be in charge of their expression.

You'll become weary...weary of the day-after-day routine...weary of seeing no improvement...weary of seeing the other person improve one day and having your hope rekindled that there may be improvement only to have the next day be a replica of other difficult days...weary of hearing the same words and complaints you've heard or said countless times before...weary of receiving your loved one's anger and irritation and yet another apology...weary of doctors not being able to give either of you the help or hope you're looking for.

This is why you will need some time to yourself as well as with others and the Lord. You need replenishment. You won't be able to do it all.

A Sometimes Subtle Danger

Dealing with the ill person in a way that makes him or her "less than you," perhaps not your equal, can creep in. Remember, even though your loved one is ill, he or she is not inferior or deficient. The person has an identity apart from the illness. The one you're caring for is still a complete person. Show equality by asking for his (or her) opinion rather than making decisions for him. Don't do anything he's capable of.

Space is another factor in caring for others. You will need your own space, and so will the person who is sick. Another word for this is "boundaries." One wife describes her years of helping:

> I've been in a helping situation for about 13 years, and we've been married for 15 years. Prior to marriage, my husband didn't have any disabilities. What he has now was the result of a very severe reaction to anesthesia after surgery. Coming out of that he had amnesia, couldn't talk, and was physically agitated so he tore both rotator cuffs in his shoulders, dislodging all the

work they'd done in his surgery on his neck. He didn't know anything. He was in ICU for five days and began to pull out of it. The result was neurological damage and difficulty with his cognitive ability to think things through.

He had surgery on his neck again and on both rotator cuffs. He had short-term memory damage. He has times when he has no recollection of some things he had learned before. Some days he is unsteady and unaware. Sometimes he has gotten lost in the neighborhood. He's better now. These episodes are rare. He wasn't able to go back to work so his depression escalated. Then his daughter was killed, and this set him back again.

The way this has impacted me personally is that it's made me stronger. I've learned that life deals you some things you never expect, so you have to trust God to get you through them. I think there are a lot of times when you wonder why, and I know there are no easy answers to that. It makes me more compassionate to others, but I don't have the energy to give to others. I feel so overwhelmed myself.

I'm weary. I'm worn out. I've had to resign some expectations I had when I got married. We never expected these things to happen. Our dreams have changed. If we have plans, we usually cancel them since he feels so bad much of the time. We've become isolated—not by design, but it's just the way it is. Some of our projects get put on hold and never get addressed. I never planned on being the main breadwinner. He just can't work so I feel blessed by this job, but I can't be as effective as I want because of all the work at home and some of my own depression.

First of all, be aware you can't do everything for the other person. If you try to, you'll burn out. You can't always be around, and you can't always be doing something for someone. If you try, how will you meet your own needs? Who else can do what you do for your loved one? When I ask those two questions of those who help sufferers, the most common answers are "no one" or "I wish I knew." It's true that others who help may do it differently than your way, and they may not give the time that you give. But let them help! Who have you asked? And who have you asked to help you come up with a list of possible helpers? The more people involved, the more the load is lightened for each person. But remember to consult the one you're helping.

Watch out for identifying too closely with the other's pain or fear. You may take them on yourself, and that won't help anyone. What does the person want you to do? Did he (or she) ask or did you just jump in? Perhaps the person suffering needs some time alone. Why not ask?[2] Here is another true story:

> At first my husband was very self-sufficient in our marriage. He had multiple sclerosis and had already outlived his doctor's guestimates. I was grieving well in advance, even before we married, not for the current situation of his death, but for what was coming down the road in the future with his illness. There was a lot of preknowledge of the disease, but when we were first married my husband didn't require much help. He was still working full time and he was driving. He was fine on his own for the first two years. Everything with his MS progressed slowly, which was a blessing for us. However, once he got a symptom it never went away.

> I stepped into his life as a helper gradually. I began to accumulate tasks. Little by little, over time, I became more involved. He went from walking with a cane to a wheelchair to an electric cart to a fully motorized wheelchair. Every time I saw a change, we grieved it together. It made it easier but also difficult. It seemed like our grieving was never over. Maybe it was hard because I was the female and able-bodied, and he was the male and needed help. But he was gracious about it. But as a couple, every place he was in his illness, so was I. Really, in a sense, I too had MS. When your spouse can't do some things anymore, neither can you. It's very hard to be a nurse and a wife or a nurse and a husband because it changes the role. It's being more of a mother— and a mother and wife don't go together. One of the best things for us was realizing that we needed help in the home. This was life-changing for us when we got some additional help.

> I was used to getting him up in the morning, showering him, dressing him, and feeding him. Then I would get myself ready

and leave for work a little after 6:00. Before we got help I was exhausted, worn out, and one time I pulled a muscle in my back and for two months I had a limp. I felt a hundred years old. Some days I felt like I just couldn't do this anymore. When we obtained help it took me out of the role of nurse for the most part, and that was very important. I was back in the role of wife. We had help for three-and-a-half years.

We had an age difference of 17 years, and he had MS as well. He died at 51. When I look back on it, I think I was really depressed—not relationally, but because we were dealing with a lot and he was getting progressively worse. I think it was harder than I realized sometimes. When a load gets heavier a little at a time, you don't always notice it. In some ways I felt less feminine, less female, because our physical relationship diminished over time. I also gained weight. Part of the physical relationship just died of—well, mentally and physically. At a young age some of the sexual part of my life ended.

I think there were many things that gave me the strength to continue on. I know beyond a shadow of a doubt that it was God's plan for me to marry my husband, even with his chronic illness. I never questioned that at all. It was God's plan no matter how long we would have together. I loved it. We only had ten years but thought we would have more. I had the benefit of knowing in advance that his disease would be fatal, whereas many don't. When I was 23 I had to ask myself, "Is this the man I want to live with the rest of my life even if he can't do anything for me or ever take out the trash or can't work? Is this who I want?" It was a very definite yes. So I never questioned my decision. There were times when I was pulling my hair out and felt I was going crazy, especially before we got help in the house. But I wasn't going to leave the marriage. Dave was worth it, and he was worthy of being taken care of. He was a rare man. It's hard to explain what an incredible man he was.

I guess the advice I would give to others is to talk to others who are in the same helper situation. This is essential. You can't do it by yourself. And if at all possible, get help to give yourself a break. As time goes on, you take on more, and you're often not aware of how much of a load you're carrying. It accumulates. Getting help was life changing. And don't let guilt take hold when you can't do something anymore.

What can you do to help? Listen and then listen again. You can listen even when the other person's not talking. Sometimes he's not able to talk, but your attentive presence lets your friend or family member know you're there to listen. Let him know you want to hear what he's feeling when he's up to talking about it.

If the ill person is devastated or coming apart at the seams or sitting there depressed, you can't make him feel better or fix the problem. When people try, it's often to help them feel useful and relieve their own anxiety about the loved one in this state. Remember, you can never be all you want to be or all the other wants you to be for him.[3]

You will be hurt at times since some of what you offer or do will be rejected. Because you haven't experienced this chronic illness, your loved one may feel uncomfortable with you while at the same time needing your help. In your heart and mind, give him permission not to be as he was. He won't be. If something is said or done that offends you, remind yourself that he isn't who he was. You may wonder, *Did I say something wrong? Am I off base?* The answer is probably no. You're dealing with unpredictability. You're all right.

You may be tempted at times to set your loved one straight spiritually. You might hear statements such as, "I thought I could count on God, but even He let me down" or "How could a loving God let something like this illness happen?" or "I think I'm losing my faith in God. I can't even pray anymore." Squelch your desire to start quoting Bible verses, give him a book, or try to provide answers. Be glad you're hearing where he is spiritually. Respond with a simple, "Yes, what's happened doesn't make much sense, does it? It's hard to understand. I wish I had an answer for you," or just listen and reflect.

There will be times when he (or she) may not want you around. If you sense that might be the case, ask, "What would be more comfortable for you at this time: for me to be here with you or for me to give you some space? I'm okay with either option." If your presence isn't needed, say, "I'll check back with you another time to see what I can do to assist you." Your positive tone of voice is essential.

One of the best ways to help another is to supply encouragement. Scripture has much to say about this. Proverbs 12:25 AMP says, "Anxiety in a man's heart weighs it down, but an encouraging word makes it glad." First Thessalonians 5:11 AMP says, "Encourage (admonish, exhort) one another and edify (strengthen and build up) one another, just as you are doing."

The *American Heritage Dictionary* has one of the better definitions of "encourage": "a tendency or disposition to expect the best possible outcome, or to dwell on the most hopeful aspect of a situation." When this is your attitude or perspective, you'll be able to encourage your loved one. Encouragement is recognizing the other person as having worth and dignity. It means paying attention when she is sharing with you.

Hebrews 10:25 says, "Let us encourage one another." "Encourage" here means to keep someone on her feet who, if left to herself, would collapse. Your encouragement serves like the concrete pilings of a structural support. This is needed when someone struggles with chronic illness.

Another very helpful idea is to look at your helping role as a ministry. Involvement and empathy are the scriptural basis for helping. Empathy is one of the most important commodities for helping. It's viewing the situation through the other person's eyes, feeling as he (or she) feels. The scriptural admonition to bear one another's burdens in Galatians 6:2 and to rejoice with those who rejoice and weep with those who weep in Romans 12:15 is empathy. And when you're called upon to help with chronic illness, empathy is essential.

Even with empathy, you won't and can't fully understand what the person with a chronic illness is going through. But communicate to the person the understanding you do have in such a manner that he realizes you've picked up on his feelings and behavior. Try to see with his eyes what his world is like. It's like being able to see another person's pain, to understand what underlies that pain, and to communicate this understanding to the person. Can you do this? Probably not completely, and it does take practice. But keep at it and be patient.

Be open to God's leading. Father Mychal Judge, who died in the 9/11 tragedy, put it well:

> Lord, take me where You want me to go,
> Let me meet whom You want me to meet.

Help me to say what You want me to say.
And keep me from getting in Your way![4]

Why not ask your loved one if he (or she) would like you to pray with him or for him? Don't be intrusive, and don't pray long. Keep it brief but sensitive. If you have the opportunity to pray for someone in the midst of deep difficulty, such as chronic illness, see it as a privilege. I have seen some people offer to pray because they don't know what to say or they're uncomfortable with silence. And some pray in an effort to fix or convict the person prayed for. The primary motivation for prayer is to *bring the suffering person to God and His resources* and to ask God for help. What's the best way to pray with the one you care about? Let us draw on what Dr. Gordon MacDonald suggests on praying for those in difficulty. He says there are five kinds of prayers people need as an intervention during times of difficulty.

1. *Give a prayer of encouragement. Encourage* also means to press courage into someone. *Discourage* means to suck courage out of him. Your hope, your courage, your belief in her and the future can be transferred to the other. Ask for God to encourage your friend, to give her strength and courage. You might share with her how precious she is in God's sight. You could read a Scripture such as Ephesians 1:4-6 to her:

> Long ago, even before he made the world, God loved us and chose us in Christ to be holy and without fault in his eyes. His unchanging plan has always been to adopt us into his own family by bringing us to himself through Jesus Christ. And this gave him great pleasure. So we praise God for the wonderful kindness he has poured out on us because we belong to his dearly loved Son (NLT).

A prayer might be, "Oh God, [my friend] means so much to me and to you. I believe as you do that she has the ability and the strength to carry on in the midst of this difficulty. Give her a clear mind, a peaceful mind, and your guidance."

When a person questions whether or not God cares for her, I have shared portions of this song, an adaptation of Zephaniah 3:14,17 and Psalm 54:2,4:

And the Father will dance over you in joy!
He will take delight in whom He loves.
Is that a choir I hear singing the praises of God?
No, the Lord God Himself is exulting over you in song!
And He will joy over you in song.
My soul will make its boast in God,
For He has answered all my cries.
His faithfulness to me is as sure as the dawn of a new day.
Awake my soul, and sing.
Let my spirit rejoice in God.
Sing, O daughter of Zion, with all of your heart.
Cast away fear and you have been restored.
Put on the garment of praise as on a festival day.
Join with the Father in glorious, jubilant song.
God rejoices over you in song![5]

2. Another prayer is the *prayer of restoration*. This is for the one who has failed or thinks he has failed. Often those with chronic illness see themselves as failures. She has nothing left and is exhausted. Her illness has overwhelmed her. She needs someone to pray and restore a sense of grace in her life. Perhaps it's as simple as "Lord, just fill [my friend] with hope for today and tomorrow. May she be secure in your arms" or "Lord, help my friend to know she is loved."

[Gordon] prayed for a friend in this way:

> O Lord God, here's my friend whom I've come to love. You know how much she's hurting today. Lord, I know that she's fearful. I know that she's in physical pain. Lord, she needs something from you that no human being can give her. She needs new power in her life. She needs new courage in her life. She needs to know that tomorrow can be brighter than anything that's been in the past. Lord, she needs the kind of strength that only heaven can give. So, Lord, would you take my friend today? I put my hands on her so you know who she is. Would you [help] my friend today and bring healing to her broken life?[6]

3. A third kind of prayer is the *prayer of affirmation*. That's the prayer in which you recognize something in the other that she cannot see in

herself: *"Lord, I thank you for the way my friend is making such good decisions this past week and the way she continues to. We see what you are doing in her life."* When you pray a prayer of affirmation of your friend, you are building value and confidence that God wants her to have. In doing this you're a "balcony person." You're leaning out of the balcony and saying, "Yes, you can do it. You're capable. See what you've already done!" Be affirming in both your prayers and your comments.

4. There is also *a prayer of blessing,* in which you pronounce upon another person what you know is God's purpose and will for him. You find this within the Scriptures again and again. *"The Lord bless you and keep you; the Lord make his face shine upon you and be gracious to you; the Lord turn his face toward you and give you peace"* (Numbers 6:24-26).

What could you say?

> Blessed be the God and Father of our Lord Jesus Christ. May He bless you with _____ .

> May the Lord bless you and keep you strong…

> May the Lord give you hope that will neither cause despair nor disappoint…

5. Last is the *prayer of intercession.* This is called for when the other is so weak and needy that you need to stand between her and God, praying on her behalf. In John 17, Jesus intercedes for His disciples. At times we are called to pray for others. You will know what is needed as you listen to what your friend says. You could pray the following:

> Father, sometimes events intrude into our lives that bring distress and discouragement. Use your Word and the work of your Holy Spirit to lift this from [my friend] and bring comfort. I thank you in advance for doing this. In Jesus' name I pray.

Or you could pray:

> Dear God, my friend needs the Holy Spirit as the Great Comforter at this moment to overcome the pain and distress. Help her.

Be simple in your prayers. Be short. Be sincere. And if you promise to pray later, write yourself a reminder so you are faithful. Also let the person know you've been praying. You will never fully understand the power and effects of prayer in your hurting friend's life.

How the Church Can Help

In the process of writing this book we asked many people, "How can the church minister to people with chronic illness?" Here are a number of responses.

> "I think that each church needs support groups as well as a mentoring program in which someone who has had an illness for some time would reach out to those at the onset of the illness."

> "Be more understanding why I'm a 'flake' and not lay a guilt trip on me that I don't attend church or Bible studies on a regular basis. I'm tired of being asked if I'm better 'this week.' I want to say that I'm never going to be better, but that makes people uncomfortable. So I just smile…and it all starts over the next week…and I'm embarrassed that I'm a 'flake'…I am honest with my close friends, just not the 'Hi, how are you?' people at church."

> "For me it's practical—a comfy place to sit during the service. Sometimes I sit on the couch in the foyer where the service is shown on TV, but then I feel like a 'slacker'!"

> "We need prayer teams and some visitation. Not expecting chronic illness sufferers to be in church every Sunday, keeping us off committees, and not expecting us to reach out to others when we cannot."

> "Recognize that God does not heal everyone the same way. He has given doctors knowledge and wisdom to deal with certain illnesses with drugs, surgery, and therapy. Even while Jesus walked in human form, there were lepers, lame, blind, suffering people He didn't heal. There are people suffering all around us who

are silenced by shame and despair. And some will go on suffering, but God can use even that for His purposes. We just need to be supportive."

"And of course for those who need it...physical help...cook a meal...drive to church...do their laundry...make sure they have funds for necessary pain medication. (That's a big one. Many do not)."

"I would like to be greeted with 'I'm happy to see you,' or 'I'm glad you could make it,' or some such thing instead of 'How are you?' I never know how to answer that and be honest. I either pretend I didn't hear the question or say some vague thing like 'I could be better,' to which people respond, 'So could I.' I don't want to invite a discussion on how I am."

"Unconditional love and acceptance. Don't treat us as if we are different. We aren't. Don't baby us. (Although sometimes hearing those 'poor baby' comments...and a cup of hot cocoa... can work wonders!) *Hold us accountable to glorify and serve God within the limitations He has allowed.* Encourage us to help others who are suffering. Don't count us out of anything. Find or make a place for us. (Like don't expect us to sign up for the 'walk-a-thon' or 'paint party,' but ask us to make the calls, collect funds, etc.). Pay attention to our gifts and encourage us to use them. When we have to withdraw a bit...leave us alone. If we let you down...tell us...but forgive us. Help us do better the next time. Don't talk about our illness to others. It's our stuff...and it should be our decision when and if we choose to tell others about it. Realize that sometimes we will show up and be in pain...and it sort of rules. We may be a bit distracted... or even irritable. Don't take it personally, but do tell us if we take it out on someone else."

Your Help Is Vital

Your loved one doesn't need pity. He (or she) needs empathy. He may dislike or resent that he needs help. He needs your belief in him and your encouragement. Each day ask yourself how you might feel, how you might behave, and what you might say if you had the chronic illness.

One of the ways you can be an advocate is educating other friends and family members about this illness and how to respond and help. Many will tend to avoid the ill person, and their withdrawal can be very painful to the suffering one. And often others avoid the person because they don't know what to say or do. Why not help them?

Living *with*
Chronic Illness

E veryone with a chronic illness has his (or her) own story. We listened to the stories of scores of people in preparation for this book. Throughout the chapters we've shared portions of many of them. In this chapter we present several in their entirety. They are responding to a survey we took. We have done some slight editing for readability. As you read these stories you will discover you are not alone in your experiences and feelings. We hope you will identify with what these individuals share and be encouraged to persevere in your illness or as a person who cares for someone suffering from chronic illness.

❧

I Refuse to Worry

In 1996 I was diagnosed with Chronic fatigue syndrome (CFS) because of chronic fatigue and pain. Lab tests didn't show any apparent problem, even though I was hardly able to get out of bed and do the typical daily duties of mothering. I was about 40 years old, and I knew that something was wrong—very wrong. Thyroid tests, blood work, etc., proved okay, it seemed. My gynecologist refused to believe I was premenopausal, even though my periods were very light. This left me with the need to research my symptoms on the Internet and in books.

Later, having more tests and after learning a lot on the Internet about fibromyalgia, CFS, thyroid issues, and lupus, the doctors seemed to believe me and saw some obvious problems. I was then diagnosed with lupus (the doctors said I have it, but I don't). Another doctor started me on thyroid medication for T-4 but not T-3 (they said I didn't need T-3). My problem with my thyroid is Hashimotus, an autoimmune form of hypothyroid, so it can change from time to time making my health harder to control. In a few years my periods disappeared. Finally my gynecologist said I was in menopause, about 15 years too early. I then had an ultrasound on my ovaries, and they couldn't find any—they had completely dried up! This resulted in a diagnosis of premature ovarian failure. So now we knew I needed some kind of hormones. I continued to research on the Internet and learned so much about others with similar problems. The hormones I wasn't getting and the low thyroid had done my body in. My doctors were somewhat helpful, but I had to learn and ask and beg them to help me in some of the areas they weren't familiar with. They just kept saying my tests were okay.

The diagnosis of lupus really scared me. I couldn't believe it. I'd always heard such bad things about it. All my life I've had allergies and extra-sensitive skin reactions to lotions. I always thought my body was a little odd. The years before my problems started I had a lot of energy and was very involved with church responsibilities and active in my boys' classrooms, sports activities, gardening, and playing tennis. Now I had lost control of the usual daily stuff that most people take for granted.

I could see that I wasn't a healthy person, and my life and my family's lives would be affected. It was difficult for my husband. He experienced some denial at the beginning. I was determined to learn what I could to help myself, but I knew it would be hard. I had to turn to the Lord for peace and strength. As I look back, I'm thankful that the Lord had grown my relationship with Him through this ordeal. Without the Lord I couldn't and can't meet the demands that my body requires of me. As my family and I began to simplify our lives and eat better in response to the hardship of illness, we did find blessings.

By far my greatest struggle has been not being able to keep up with life. I used to do many things and enjoy life, people, doing and giving my time. Now I'm very limited and am always behind the game. I understand this, but it is still very hard. I have to depend on the Lord to help me get the most important stuff done. So often, and especially during holidays, I just run out of energy. When I'm too busy or doing too much I can't tell what my body needs, so it starts getting weird on me. Many times I am in so much pain—intestinal problems, hormone symptoms, muscle pain, fatigue, and discouragement. Many years ago I learned I couldn't feel sorry for myself because it created other problems. So I remain positive, lower my expectations, and accept the circumstances. There are good days, and there are bad days. I can't keep my body doing what I want all the time. I feel as though I live at 75-percent normal. So I'm thankful for that. So many are worse off than me.

Another hard struggle has been with family. Not my immediate family—but extended family. They're not considerate or helpful and have zero empathy. I have an older sister, and in the many years I've had this illness, she's asked me how I felt just one time—during the early stages when I was in bed all day. My mother felt sorry for me but never helped me with meals or kids. The same with my mother-in-law. She is a "doing" person and is not relational with anyone. There was no Christian love here for me in my greatest times of need from loved ones. The Lord became my *best* Friend, and He was here for me when others weren't.

My husband has been here for me as much as a husband can be. He does have trouble remembering I can't do all the things we want to do. He is a very going and doing type of person. Through the years he's helped me with housework, etc. My boys are caring but sometimes forget mom has many problems. It's hard for them to relate. I remember when they were younger I told the Lord he was going to have to raise my boys because I physically couldn't do all I needed to do. God did such a good job!

Another hard part has been the doctors throughout the experience. They just don't know enough about hormonal and endocrine problems in women. Thankfully, the Internet has made so much information available to me through medical Websites, message boards, and forums. Some people really care about getting the truth out about health issues and what is indeed best for our bodies. I've had to teach my doctors many things, and it took longer to get to the causes than it should have. I wanted to know details about my problems rather than just treat the symptoms, as so many doctors tend to do these days. I wanted to take an alternative approach as much as possible and keep off heavy medications. I take natural hormones and supplements, thyroid medication, antihistamines, B-12 injections, Betaine HCL (my stomach doesn't make acid to break down food), enzymes, and others.

I've had caring people ask about me and understand my difficulties, but they are the minority. Yes, the church doesn't seem to understand. People are so into doing church activities and getting self-gratitude from what they do. I just wish they would learn to do less and spend more time in relationship with the Lord and do what He wants them to do. I don't compare myself to others, but it's hard not to want to do good things that require time and energy. My Lord has me right where He wants me.

It's difficult and a daily struggle to manage my body. If it isn't one thing, it's another. I can tolerate a lot of pain, but it's discouraging at times. I would like others to respect the fact that I have a disability and that it is a very humbling and alone process. Nobody seems to care because it is ongoing but not acute. Understanding chronic problems isn't easy, and the fact I just can't do whatever I want to do is difficult for people to comprehend. The fatigue part of chronic problems is mentally tough. I have to have so much mind-over-matter when my body is not working right. Also I can't do something just because I want to—I have to be physically able. Life just isn't that easy with my condition. I think others think I'm weak and lazy—and I'm not at all!

I've felt sadness, very alone, weakened, ignored, loss of hope, no way out, alienated from normal life, disappointed a lot, discouraged, hopeless at times, empty of worth, worthless, helpless, ashamed—those are the worst emotions. Many times I've felt blessed that I have this illness because the Lord has become someone I lean on for the most simple things. He wants me to come to Him and ask for help. The Lord is my Healer so many times with even the most little things. He is always here beside me, even when no one else is. He is my Helper and my Refuge. He knows my abilities and my capabilities. He knows my heart and my motives.

I wish others would pray for me, think of me, and know that it's hard to have a chronic illness. I wish that when they ask how I am doing concerning my health they would actually listen for a bit. When my husband realizes that I am in a period of pain and fatigue, he will say he is sorry for me and he can't believe how hard it must be. When he realizes and understands that I can't get going as quickly in the morning or our plans have to be altered or changed because I can't get there, it helps. Usually I find it's the same people that show care and concern, but the majority don't give compassion. When others understand my limitations it helps. I do have some extended family—cousins and aunts—that always ask and care for me.

I think it would be helpful for the church to have support groups for chronic pain sufferers. Especially for newcomers to chronic illness. Through support groups, they learn they're not alone on this path of pain, also they can get encouragement and helpful tips. Information and doctors' names could be shared, meeting together for prayer, etc., and probably teaching the church that we need to care more about each other. Many are too busy with working, hobbies, spending money, and trying to get ahead. We need each other and at some point we all need love, compassion, and encouragement. I haven't really felt God was punishing me with this chronic illness for sins, etc. Maybe some people do, but I am not hung up on that. Rather, I feel special to the Lord, that He wanted more of me in right relationship to Him.

I wish people understood that chronic illness is sometimes debilitating physically. I cannot do in the church as I would like when it comes to serving.

What have I done to be hopeful and survive? I think always being aware of my need for balance by not doing too much and not eating the wrong things that make my symptoms worse. I try to maintain steady discipline in leading a balanced life even though I can't really achieve it. When I think I have a balance, then sure enough I go through a bad spell. I realize again I am just not a normal person. Staying in close contact with the Lord and reading the Bible—this is my *best* help, but sometimes I can't do this. But I can always talk to God.

I refuse to worry and fret about the future. Sometimes I think, *What will I do when I am older or this or that?* This is the negative energy I have to get rid of. The Lord is my Great Helper in all things. He reminds me when I've wandered away from Him how much I need Him for every little thing, even what I eat and how much I eat. I haven't asked, "Why me?" God has renewed my walk with Him to levels I couldn't have had if I were independently living my own busy and active life. I have seen the Lord bless me and my family so many times for some of our sacrifices with this illness. The sickness has brought us much closer in our relationship with each other. I don't fear the future with my health because the Lord gives me peace.

I need to strive to meet each day with my wants and needs. I take it one day at a time. The Lord has shown me so many times His healing power. I'm amazed at His care for me. I pray this for others who endure similar health problems. It's hard when you know the illness is here to stay, but God is bigger than any of our problems.

Yes, It's a Real Disease

I have Charcot-Marie-Tooth disease, which is now classified as a form of muscular dystrophy. It comes in different types. What I have affects my lungs and muscle tone. The doctors weren't aware I had this type until this year. I also have another type, which I was diagnosed with when I was about 21. Now I'm in my fifties. When I experienced my first intense episode, I stopped breathing...and then my heart stopped. I was in the process of a long hospitalization and was moved from one hospital to another because the doctors were baffled by my condition. A medical student fresh out of school was the one who actually diagnosed me! This was in the seventies, and they had just come up with a name for the disease. Back then they didn't narrow it down by the types we have today. My type is very aggressive, and it affects me from the hips down. I've worn leg braces for 35 years. My arms are affected as well, from the clavicle area to the fingertips. This disease is progressive. It used to only progress in the summer because of the heat, but now it progresses all the time.

I worked through my mid forties. I'm an RN. I preferred neurosurgery intensive care since it challenged my brain the most. I've done everything from burn trauma to heart transplants, but neuro was an area that kept me mentally enthralled and challenged. I worked with some of the best surgeons in the world.

Now my primary struggle is finances. I knew at a young age I would be disabled, so I tried to plan for it financially. I was told that by the time I was 30 I would be a paralytic, but I'm still walking. I worked 15 years after I turned 30. I had planned financially as well as I could and did well, but I was taken in a personal identity theft by a family member. I lost most of what I'd saved.

Other than financial, I'm faced by a lot of discrimination, even in the medical field. I'm an intelligent person and can be gainfully employed using my mind, but what stands in my way are people. When I knew I couldn't work, the neurologist I went to see wouldn't describe on the forms specifically what I actually had but wrote something general. What I have is an actual disease, but his response was, "Well, maybe you have a problem." When he asked me why I couldn't work, I said, "The pain was just phenomenal—I couldn't do my 12- to 16-hour shift anymore." His response was there's no reason I should be having pain. His philosophy was, "If you can smile, you're not in pain." At one time I had five broken bones in my leg, and I never said a thing while I was worked on. I also had torn ligaments. I developed a high tolerance to pain so I could continue working. I had to. When people see me walking with my brace, they tend to think the disability isn't that great.

Other people, such as those in my small group at church, have been very supportive. They know not to offer me assistance unless I ask for it. But they also go out of their way for me. My own family members don't understand how strenuous it is for me to do simple things anymore, such as climb a ladder or walk up two steps without a railing. People will hand me things and think I have them, but my hands don't hold onto them. It's like I have body parts that have their own minds. I am much worse than people think, and I do my best to make each day all right. But at the same time I see no reason to prolong my life. This upsets others, but if I'm seriously injured or gravely ill, I don't see a need to go on. I know with God there's a better life waiting for me. Here on earth I'm making do with the best I have, but I refuse to let my misery continue on if I get into a worse situation.

I wish others would give me an opportunity to work and prove my worth. My mind is sharp, and I can work. But what jobs are offered to me, if anything, are measly and don't use my abilities.

When I first came to Jesus I didn't know about my disease. I just knew that my legs hurt so much almost all the time, and people would put their hands on me and pray: "Make this illness go away." When it didn't, they said, "It's of the devil. You have the devil in you, and you're not trying to get it out." That made me feel terrible. I understand that their intent was good, but the fact that my illness didn't go away was actually more devastating to them than it was to me. I was learning to live with my disability and learning to conquer what I needed to so my life would be as normal as possible. If by chance a miracle were to happen and I would lose this disability, this disease, and I was totally normal, I honestly wouldn't know how to act or to be. I would be more scared of being normal than being how I am today. I'm afraid if I could do normal person things I'd not have to depend on God…so I might lose my connection with Him. And I don't think I'm the only person who feels this way.

What has helped me continue to survive with this illness is seeing what I have as a day-by-day struggle—actually an hour-by-hour struggle. I look at every day as simply something to get through, trying to be positive in my outlook yet realistic. I become quite annoyed when people say, "Oh, it will get better" or "Don't think about it." Well, I'd love to not think about it. I have my best interest in mind, but at the same time I'm not looking for a miracle from God.

The older I get, the harder it gets. When I was in my teens or twenties, I never pictured that I would be 55 years old. I knew the side effects of this disease would eventually kill me. My disease has stopped two careers, and I'm searching for a third. Having God has made a difference.

⌇

Fear Not

I have a disease called polycythemia vera. I was diagnosed two years ago. It's an acquired disorder of the bone marrow that causes the over-production of white blood cells, red blood cells, and platelets. It is a rare disorder that occurs more frequently in men than women and rarely in patients under age 40. The exact cause is unknown. The danger with polycythemia is that having too many blood cells thickens the blood and can cause blood clots and other problems.

I was shocked and scared when I found out about my illness. It was initially discovered during a routine blood test. I didn't know anything was wrong, but I was called right away to come back to the doctor for further testing. The doctor told me I most likely had a rare genetic disease or cancer. As you can imagine, neither diagnosis sounded good. They referred me to a hematologist/oncologist for further testing.

I had to wait almost a month to get in to the specialist, and during that time I went through a variety of emotions. I tried to remain strong and trust the Lord, but I was also consumed with fear and worry. It was not an easy month. Once I saw a blood specialist, he tested me for a rare blood disorder.

Thankfully what I have can be controlled with treatment. Controlled— but not cured. The good news, of course, was that I would have an average life expectancy as long as I have my blood levels monitored regularly and continue treatment. When I heard that, I was so relieved and thankful to not have cancer! I praised God that they caught the disorder before something catastrophic happened. I was taking medication that could have increased the risk of blood clots, so I was immediately switched to a different one.

One of the greatest struggles has been all the testing and treatment. I am very fearful of needles, and medical professionals have always had problems finding my veins. As I have a blood disorder, you can imagine how many times I've been poked to be tested. I have had a series of very painful and scary tests including a bone marrow biopsy to rule out cancer. The treatment for the level of polycythemia I have is routine phlebotomies, where they take a large quantity of my blood to reduce my blood cell count. This has been very difficult as the needle is very large and painful. They usually have to "try" for a vein multiple times before getting one.

The other byproduct of this disorder is that my doctor is very concerned about pregnancy. I am 25 and have been told to use multiple methods of birth control as pregnancy would be very dangerous for both me and a baby. I've been told that once my husband and I want to start trying I'll need to be very carefully monitored by a doctor. The reason for this is that increased hormones in my body can increase the risk of blood clots. In addition, my thick blood may make it impossible for blood to make it through the umbilical cord for a baby.

In order to get pregnant and keep a baby, I will have to have additional treatments, including daily injections of a blood thinner. This has been a great struggle because my husband and I had planned for a number of children. We've had to deal with the reality that we may not be able to have as many as we would have liked…if any at all. I'm thankful that I do know about this ahead of time and that we didn't find out about this until something serious happened to a baby or to me. But at the same time I worry about getting pregnant, worry if we will ever have children, and worry about what will happen when we try.

To mitigate the worry, I focus on remembering the Lord has a plan and purpose for my life, no matter how long it may be and no matter what happens. I know I can trust the Lord in all things, even though I don't always do a great job of giving Him my worry and fear. There is a scripture that has been very powerful for me: "We rejoice in the hope of the glory of God. Not only so, but we also rejoice in our sufferings, because we know that suffering produces perseverance; perseverance, character; and character, hope" (Romans 5:2-4).

I've been blessed by the great doctors I've had through this experience. The doctor that originally found my abnormal blood test wasn't my regular doctor. This had to be of the Lord because my regular doctor was quite frustrating. She didn't listen to me and often seemed to prescribe medicine just to get me out of her office. The doctor filling in for her was just what I needed. He was direct and to the point, but he was also very understanding about how scared I was. He told me what was wrong and told me the plan. He was open to hearing and addressing all the questions I had. He also told me I could call with any additional questions I might have while I waited to see the specialist. He was a God-send! I did need to call him while I waited. Again he was patient and understanding. When I did get in to see the oncologist/hematologist I was again blessed, as this doctor was also kind and patient. He reminded me of my grandfather, which put me at ease. Through all the testing he has been gentle and understanding. He understands that pregnancy is part of my life plan, and he has done additional studying and research to learn all he can about polycythemia and pregnancy (it's rare for women of childbearing age to have this disorder). I see him every two months, and he continues to be helpful. He knows how much trouble I have when they do the phlebotomies, so he takes care to have his best nurse do the procedures. I have to say I haven't always had the best doctors, but the Lord has provided wonderful physicians for me throughout this experience.

Because my body expends energy to produce too many blood cells, my overall energy level is sapped. In addition, the treatment makes me anemic. I am also supposed to keep to a low iron diet (which, believe it or not, helps slow the production of blood cells). As a result of those two things, I get very tired near the end of the day, and I *need* to get at least eight hours of sleep. Another symptom of my disorder is chronic migraines. I have suffered from migraines and headaches for years. On the one hand it's nice to know what's causing these headaches since they can be very painful and debilitating. I think for me the final pain is often emotional. Living with a chronic illness that can't be cured is daunting. Wondering if I will be able to have children is also very painful.

I think I have experienced every emotion under the sun as a result of this disease. I've been scared, sad, angry, depressed, grateful, miserable, joyful, tired, and hungry for answers.

My family and friends' love and support have been most helpful during this whole process. Several of my family members have stepped up to be there for me during the toughest times. I've had family members offer to go with me to treatments and have followed through. My boss has been wonderfully understanding as well. On days when I have to go for my treatment we have it worked out so I don't have to come back to work as it is emotionally and physically draining. I just can't express enough how wonderful my friends and especially my family have been. I am thankful for the responses of others. Overall, I think my family and friends have been very supportive and that has helped a lot. Just knowing people love and care about me makes a huge difference.

There have been a few painful experiences. People don't always know how to respond to someone with a chronic illness. Most don't understand what I go through in terms of getting the phlebotomies—especially if giving blood isn't an issue for them.

When I was waiting for a diagnosis, everyone was saying that everything was going to be okay, but they weren't living in my head. They couldn't understand how scared I was. It seemed insensitive and flippant for people to just say that everything was going to be okay, and that I was worrying for nothing. How could they know?

Another problem is, like most anything else: out of sight, out of mind. Initially people were very helpful and concerned, but now often it's like nothing ever happened. People don't check in to see how I'm feeling or coping. It feels like they've forgotten I deal with this on a daily basis… or at least it feels like they don't care.

I think it's easy to ignore or forget that people are hurting when you can't see it. I also feel like sometimes churchgoers give pat answers, such as "just pray more," and often that feels insincere. I know I need to pray more often when I feel worried or fearful, but it seems that is often the only answer from the church. Instead of a pat answer, it would be helpful to be supported and joined in prayer, which would validate my worries and fears. Some people avoid people who are hurting because they don't know what to say.

I think at this point I know what I have to deal with. I know this is the life I've been blessed with and the life that I live. It isn't helpful to live in denial or to be scared all the time. Instead, I embrace that this is who I am and that God has a greater purpose for this in my life. I may not know or understand that purpose, but I pray God will use this for His glory. I remember that He is here with me. I am not alone in this! He blessed me with wonderful family, friends, and doctors. When this ordeal first started, my brother gave me a ring that says "Fear Not," and that is how I choose to live. Having a positive attitude is a choice, and that is what I try to choose every day.

❧

Supported by Love

I have systemic lupus—my body is allergic to its own cells. When I get sick, my body attacks itself. I was diagnosed at age 14. That was hard because I was a sophomore in high school. I came home from cheerleading camp and had this butterfly rash on my face, which is really common for those with lupus. I'd had lupus for some time, but I didn't know it. I guess I had it even as a young child. I would come home from elementary school and take naps—and that's not normal. On Sunday after church, if I wanted to go back to church in the evening, I'd have to take a three-hour nap to be rested enough. My parents and I knew something was wrong, but we didn't know what. I've always slept a lot. Sleep is essential. And rest has always been critical for me, but I also want to have time to live! Fortunately, I had knowledgeable doctors from the beginning.

My biggest adjustment has been that I can't be out in the sun. That's difficult. When I was younger, it was hard because my friends went to the beach. I was also a lifeguard for a couple of summers. I majored in physical education in college, which probably wasn't smart. I thought I could beat the odds and show I could do something against what I had.

I need much more rest than the average person, and when I get sick I can be down for weeks at a time. Wintertime is usually more difficult.

When I was younger it was harder for me than now because back then people didn't know what lupus was. I was the first to be diagnosed with lupus in Orange County, California. I had the rash on my face, lost my hair, and people made fun of me. I always felt left out because I couldn't do what my friends could do. Some people were understanding, but some were cruel. As an adult I find that some people don't understand, especially at my work. They see my seemingly healthy outward appearance and can't get it that I'm sick on the inside. I don't want to use this disease as a crutch, and I never have. But people don't understand why others get over sicknesses so much faster than I do. My body can't fight illness off very well.

Because I sleep a lot, people ask, "Why do you go to bed so early?" If I don't go to bed at eight o'clock, I can't get up the next day. I can't do what everybody else can do, and when I try I pay for it dearly. I've learned I have to manage my life.

This disease is really hard on the family. My husband does 100 percent of the heavy housework at home. He's carrying two or three times the load most husbands do. I don't have the energy, and if I don't get down time, I crash.

Since this is an autoimmune disease and people are so conscious of AIDS, some wonder if it's contagious. They don't want to be near me because they might catch it. The brave ones ask, "Can I catch it from you?" I'm not a doctor so I don't know if I can explain lupus properly to them.

Fortunately, I've had good experiences with my doctors. My immediate family has been very supportive. My husband has been here for me all the time, and he doesn't baby me. He uses a tough-love approach but keeps after me not to overdo, which is my tendency. And the churches we've been to have been supportive in practical ways—taking me to doctors and providing meals. Even people I work with have been helpful. Some days I was too sick to drive home and someone would take me while someone else would drive my car to my house.

I believe each church needs a support group as well as mentoring programs, in which someone who has had an illness for some time would reach out to those at the onset of their illnesses.

I don't want my disease to keep me from living my life. My husband has to "tame" me down a lot, and he's always done so because I want to keep going until I collapse. I need to be my own physician because who knows me better than myself?

Alternative Treatments
for Pain Management

Research shows these therapies can ease discomfort. For more information visit the Website of the National Center for Complementary and Alternative Medicine. Loolwa Khazzoom compiled this helpful chart.[1] We've made minor adaptions, indicated by brackets.

Type	What They Help	How They Work	Examples
Movement-Based Therapies Physical exercises and practices	Musculoskeletal pain, joint pain, and lower-back pain	By strengthening muscles supporting joints, improving alignment, and releasing endorphins	**Physical therapy:** Specialized movements to strengthen weak areas of the body, often through resistance training **Yoga:** [The stretching and poses only, *not* the religious aspects] **Pilates:** A resistance regimen that strengthens core muscles **Tai chi:** A slow, flowing Chinese practice that improves balance **Feldenkrais:** A therapy that builds efficiency of movement

Type	What They Help	How They Work	Examples
Nutritional and Herbal Remedies Food choices and dietary supplements (ask your doctor before using supplements)	All chronic pain but especially abdominal discomfort, headaches, and inflammatory conditions such as rheumatoid arthritis	By boosting the body's natural immunity, reducing pain-causing inflammation, soothing pain, and decreasing insomnia	**Anti-inflammatory diet:** A Mediterranean eating pattern high in whole grains, fresh fruits, leafy vegetables, fish, and olive oil **Omega-3 fatty acids:** Nutrients abundant in fish oil and flaxseed that reduce inflammation in the body **Ginger:** A root that inhibits pain-causing molecules **Turmeric:** A spice that reduces inflammation **MSM:** Methylsulfonylmethane, a naturally occurring nutrient that helps build bone and cartilage

Type	What They Help	How They Work	Examples
Mind-Body Medicine Using the powers of the mind to produce changes in the body	All types of chronic pain	By reducing stressful (and, hence, pain-inducing) emotions such as panic and fear, and by refocusing attention on subjects other than pain	**Meditation:** Focusing the mind on something specific (such as breathing or repeating a word or phrase) to quiet it. [As Christians, we recommend focusing on God and His principles.] **Guided imagery:** Visualizing a particular outcome or scenario with the goal of mentally changing one's physical reality **Biofeedback:** With a special machine, becoming alert to body processes, such as muscle tightening, to learn to control them **Relaxation:** Releasing tension in the body through exercises such as controlled breathing

Type	What They Help	How They Work	Examples
Energy Healing Manipulating the body's electrical energy...emitted by the nervous system	Pain that lingers after an injury heals, as well as pain complicated by trauma, anxiety, or depression	By relaxing the body and the mind, distracting the nervous system, producing natural painkillers	**Acupuncture:** The insertion of hair-thin needles into points along the body's meridians, or energetic pathways. [Western medicine believes the insertion points stimulate nerves, muscles, and connective tissue, boosting the activity of the body's natural painkillers and blood flow.][2]

Type	What They Help	How They Work	Examples
Physical Manipulation Hands-on massage or movement of painful areas	Musculoskeletal pain, especially lower-back and neck pain; pain from muscle underuse or overuse; and pain from adhesions or scars	By restoring mobility, improving circulation, decreasing blood pressure, and relieving stress	**Massage:** The manipulation of tissue to relax clumps of knotted muscle fiber, increase circulation, and release patterns of chronic tension **Chiropractic:** Physically moving vertebrae or other joints into proper alignment, to relieve stress **Osteopathy:** Realigning vertebrae, ribs, and other joints, as with chiropractic; osteopaths have training equivalent to that of medical doctors

Type	What They Help	How They Work	Examples
Lifestyle Changes Developing healthy habits at home and work	All types of chronic pain	By strengthening the immune system and enhancing well-being, and by reframing one's relationship to (and, thus, experience of) chronic pain	**Sleep hygiene:** Creating an optimal sleep environment to get deep, restorative rest; strategies include establishing a regular sleep-and-wake schedule and minimizing light and noise.

Positive work environment: Having a comfortable workspace and control over one's activities to reduce stress and contribute to the sense of mastery over pain.

Healthy relationships: Nurturing honest and supportive friendships and family ties to ease anxiety that exacerbate pain.

Exercise: Regular activity to build strength and lower stress |

A Pain Diary

Date/Time	Pain Level	Type of Pain	Recent Activities/Conditions	Action Taken (if any)	Results of Action Taken
Date					
Time					
Date					
Time					
Date					
Time					
Date					
Time					

Adapted from *The Chronic Pain Solution*[1]

Dietary Supplement Definitions

Choline: usually made from phenylalanine, but also widely distributed in many foods. Choline is important for normal membrane function and acetylcholine synthesis. The choline requirement for adults is 550mg per day. Foods with the highest total choline concentration (mg/100 g) are beef liver (418), chicken liver (290), eggs (251), wheat germ (152), bacon (125), dried soybeans (116), and pork (103). (This information is from the American Society for Nutritional Sciences *Journal of Nutrition* (May 2003).

Phenylalanine: animal and vegetable proteins, vegetables, and juices. It is also found in fermented food such as yogurt and miso.

Tryptophan: dairy products, beef, turkey, bananas, poultry, barley, brown rice, fish, soybeans, and peanuts.

Tyrosine: animal and vegetable proteins, vegetables, juices and fermented food such as yogurt and miso.

Vitamin B6: meat, fish, poultry, dried beans, bananas, potatoes, raisins, and dried figs, dates and prunes. (Information from the 2005 PDR Web site).[1]

Notes

Can You Relate?

1. Two Listeners, *God Calling,* A.J. Russell, ed., www.twolisteners.org, May 12, circa 1932.

Chapter 1: A World of Pain and Frustration

1. Jeffrey H. Boyd, *Being Sick Well* (Grand Rapids, MI: Baker Books, 2005), p. 8.
2. Paul J. Donoghue, Ph.D., and Mary E. Siegel, Ph.D., *Sick and Tired of Feeling Sick and Tired* (New York: W.W. Norton Co., 2000), pp. 12-13, adapted.
3. Linda Rainey Wright, *Good Days, Bad Days* (Nashville: Thomas Nelson, 1991), pp. 18-22, adapted.
4. Ibid., p. 23.
5. Sefra Kobrin Pitzele, *We Are Not Alone* (New York: Workman Publishing, 1988), p. 12, adapted.
6. Marva Dawn, *Being Well When We're Ill* (Minneapolis: Augsburg Fortress, 2008), p. 14.
7. Cheryl Register, *The Chronic Illness Experience* (Center City, MN: Hazeldon, 1987), pp. xvi-xvii, adapted.
8. Eugenie G. Wheeler and Joyce Dace-Lombard, *Living Creatively with Chronic Illness* (Ventura, CA: Pathfinder Publishing, 1989), p. 102, adapted.
9. Carl J. Charnetski and Francis X. Brennan, *Feeling Good Is Good for You* (Emmaus, PA: Rodale Books, 2001), pp. 12-21, adapted.
10. Jessie Gruman, Ph.D., *AfterShock* (New York: Walker & Co., 2007), pp. 41-43, adapted.
11. *The Lutheran Prayer Book: A Collection of Prayer and Inspiration for Every Lutheran* (Nashville: Woodbury, 1989), p. 53.

Chapter 2: The Search for a Diagnosis

1. Paul J Donoghue, Ph.D., and Mary E. Siegel, Ph.D., *Sick and Tired of Feeling Sick and Tired* (New York: W.W. Norton Co., 2000), pp. 71-76, adapted.
2. Carol Sveilich, M.A., *Just Fine* (Austin: Avid Reader Press, 2005), p. 31.
3. Donoghue and Siegel, *Sick and Tired,* p. 77.
4. Sefra Kobrin Pitzele, *We Are Not Alone* (New York: Workman Publishing, 1988), pp. 25-26, adapted.

5. Jessie Gruman, *AfterShock* (New York: Walker & Co., 2007), p. 2, adapted.

6. Kathleen Lewis, *Celebrate Life* (Atlanta: Arthritis Foundation, 1999), pp. 35-37, adapted.

7. Listed in Pitzele, *We Are Not Alone,* p. 54, adapted.

8. Sveilich, *Just Fine,* p. 14.

9. Lewis, *Celebrate Life,* pp. 40-42, adapted.

10. Ibid., n.p.

11. Nancy Davis, *Lean on Me* (New York: A Fireside Book, 2006), pp. 66-67.

12. Norman Cousins, *Anatomy of an Illness As Perceived by the Patient* (New York: W.W. Norton & Company, 2001), n.p.

13. Davis, *Lean on Me,* pp. 16, 20, 24, adapted.

14. Ibid., p. 16.

15. Jack Hayford, *Hope for the Hopeless Day* (Ventura, CA: Regal Books, 2007), pp. 11-12.

Chapter 3: The People in Your Life

1. Jessie Gruman, Ph.D., *AfterShock* (New York: Walker & Co., 2007), pp. 18-20, adapted.

2. Ibid., p. 22, adapted.

3. Ibid., p. 25, adapted.

4. Nancy Davis, *Lean on Me* (New York: A Fireside Book, 2006), pp. 16, 20, 24, adapted.

5. Lauri Edwards, *Life Disrupted* (New York: Walker and Co., 2008), p. 21, adapted.

6. Gruman, *AfterShock,* pp. 62-65, adapted.

7. Winnie Yu, *The Everything Health Guide to Fibromyalgia* (Avon, MA: Adams Media, 2006), p. 61, adapted.

8. Sefra Kobrin Pitzele, *We Are Not Alone* (New York: Workman Publishing, 1988), p. 12, adapted.

9. Gruman, *AfterShock,* pp. 111-14, adapted.

10. Michael F. Roezen, M.D., and Mehmet G. Oz, M.D., *You, the Smart Patient* (New York: Free Press, 2006), pp. 224-36, adapted.

11. Kathy Charmaz, *Good Days, Bad Days* (Brusack, NJ: Rutgers University Press, 1997), pp. 109-18, adapted.

12. Carol Sveilich, *Just Fine* (Austin: Avid Reader Press, 2005), pp. 50-56, adapted.

13. Charmaz, *Good Days,* pp. 125-29, adapted.

Chapter 4: Your Family

1. John Piper and Justin Taylor, eds., *Suffering and the Sovereignty of God* (Wheaton, IL: Crossway, 2006), pp. 156-57.

2. William July, Ph.D., and Jenny Lucy July, *A Husband, a Wife, an Illness* (Bloomington, IN: Universe Inc., 2008), pp. 4-5, adapted.

3. Julie N. Silvia, *Chronic Pain and the Family* (Cambridge: Harvard University Press, 2004), pp. 87-93, adapted.

4. Eugenie G. Wheeler and Joyce Dace-Lombard, *Living Creatively with Chronic Illness* (Ventura, CA: Pathfinder Publishing, 1989), p. 69, adapted.

5. Ibid., p. 22, adapted.

6. Ibid., p. 63, adapted.

7. Dennis C. Turk, Ph.D., and Fritz Winter, Ph.D., *The Pain Survival Guide* (Washington, D.C.: American Psychological Association, 2006), p. 101.

8. Sefra Kobrin Pitzele, *We Are Not Alone* (New York: Workman Publisher, 1985), p. 61.

9. Ibid., pp. 65-66.

10. July and July, *A Husband, a Wife, an Illness,* p. 13, adapted.

11. Ibid., pp. 16-17, adapted.

12. Chris McGonigle, *Surviving Your Spouse's Chronic Illness* (New York: Henry Holt & Co., 1999), p. 18.

13. Ibid., p. 5.

14. Ibid., p. 163.

15. Silvia, *Chronic Pain and the Family,* p. 26, adapted.

16. Ibid., pp. 30-31, adapted.

Chapter 5: The Power of Pain

1. Cheri Register, *The Chronic Illness Experience* (Center City, MN: Hazelden, 1987), p. 24.

2. Ira Byock, M.D., *The Four Things That Matter Most* (New York: Free Press, 2004), p. 59.

3. Marva Dawn, *Being Well When We're Ill* (Minneapolis: Augsburg Fortress, 2008), p. 119.

4. *The Journal of Neuroscience*, Feb. 6, adapted; Northwestern University News Center, Nov. 26, 2008.

5. National Institute of Neurological Disorders and Stroke, Nov. 14, 2002.

6. www.aarpmagazine.org, Jan./Feb. 2009, pp. 25-27.

7. Marlene Hunter, *Making Peace with Chronic Pain* (New York: Bruner/Mazell, 1996), p. 5, adapted.

8. Paul J. Donaghue, Ph.D., and Mary E. Siegel, Ph.D., *Sick and Tired of Being Sick and Tired* (New York: W.W. Norton & Co., 2000), p. 41, adapted.

9. Ibid., pp. 43-45.

10. Dennis C. Turk, Ph.D., and Frits Winter, Ph.D., *The Pain Survival Guide* (Washington, D.C.: American Psychological Association, 2006), p. 12.

11. Ibid., pp. 16-17, adapted.

12. James N. Dillard, M.D., D.C., with Leigh Ann Hirschman, *The Chronic Pain Solution* (New York: Bantam Books, 2002), p. 62.

13. Turk and Winter, *Pain Survival Guide,* p. 24, adapted.

14. Dillard with Hirschman, *Chronic Pain Solution,* p. 54, adapted.

15. Devin Starlanyl and Mary Ellen Copeland, *Fibromyalgia and Chronic Myofascial Pain* (Oakland, CA: New Harbinger Publications, Inc., 2002), p. 115.

16. Turk and Winter, *Pain Survival Guide,* p. 28, adapted.

17. William July, Ph.D., and Jamey Lacy July, *A Husband, A Wife, and an Illness* (New York: Universe, Inc., 2008), pp. 111-20, adapted.

18. John H. Selak and Steven S. Overman, M.D., M.P.V., *You Don't Look Sick* (New York: Haworth Medical Press, 2005), p. 11, adapted.

19. Ibid., p. 67.

20. Ibid., p. 35, adapted.

21. Ibid., pp. 85-93, adapted.

Chapter 6: Dealing with Loss

1. Nina Herman Donnelly, *I Never Know What to Say* (New York: Ballantine Books, 1987), p. 123, adapted.

2. Linda Noble Topf with Hal Zina Bennett, *You Are Not Your Illness* (New York: Simon & Schuster, 1995), pp. 47, 42.

3. Ibid., p. 50, adapted.

4. Eugenie G. Wheeler and Joyce Dace-Lombard, *Living Creatively with Chronic Illness* (Ventura, CA: Pathfinder Publishing, 1989), p. 62, adapted.

5. Ranyon Roy, *Chronic Pain, Loss and Suffering* (Toronto, Canada: University of Toronto, 2004), pp. 60-61, adapted.

6. Judith Viorst, *Necessary Losses* (New York: Simon & Schuster, 1986), n.p.

7. Roy, *Chronic Pain, Loss, and Suffering,* pp. 80-82, adapted.

8. Lauri Edwards, *Life Disrupted* (New York: Walker and Co., 2008), p. 227.

9. Wheeler and Dace-Lombard, *Living Creatively,* pp. 65-67, adapted.

10. Sefra Korbin Pitzele, *We Are Not Alone* (New York: Thompson & Company, 1985), pp. 53-54, adapted.

11. Wheeler and Dace-Lombard, *Living Creatively,* p. 24.

12. Ibid., pp. 18-26, adapted.

13. *Helping a Grieving Person Recover and Say Good-Bye,* original source unknown.

14. Therese Rando, *Grieving: How to Go on Living When Someone You Love Dies* (Lexington, MA: Lexington Books, 1988), pp. 18-19, adapted.

15. Bob Deits, *Life After Loss* (Tucson: Fisher Books, 1988), p. 27, adapted.

16. Ibid., p. 28.

17. James Froelich, O.F.M. Cap, in a paper written for the "Pastoral Helping Relationship" graduate course (Loyola College, Baltimore, 1984).

18. Rando, *Grieving,* p. 19, adapted.

19. Ibid., p. 79, adapted.

20. Chris McGonigle, *Surviving Your Spouse's Chronic Illness* (New York: Henry Holt and Co., 1999), p. 20.

21. Kathleen Lewis, *Celebrate Life* (Atlanta: Arthritis Foundation, 1999), p. 27.

Chapter 7: Your Fluctuating Emotions

1. Dan B. Allender, Ph.D., and Tremper Longman, III, Ph.D., *The Cry of the Soul* (Colorado Springs: NavPress, 1994), pp. 16-34, adapted.

2. Joni Eareckson Tada and Steve Estes, *When God Weeps* (Grand Rapids, MI: Zondervan, 2000), pp. 157-58.

3. Ibid., p. 152.

4. Linda Noble Topf with Hal Zina Bennett, *You Are Not Your Illness* (New York: Simon & Schuster, 1995), pp. 32-33, adapted.

5. Ibid., p. 33.

6. Ibid., p. 60.

7. Ibid., pp. 60-61.

8. Jeanne Sega, Ph.D., *Living Beyond Fear*, taken from Topf with Bennett, *You Are Not Your Illness*, adapted.

9. Marlene Hunter, *Making Peace with Chronic Pain* (New York: Bruner/Mazell, 1996), p. 120, adapted.

10. Joseph Cooke, *Free for the Taking* (1975) was reprinted under the name *Celebration of Grace* (Grand Rapids, MI: Zondervan, 1991), pp. 109-10.

11. Noble Topf with Bennett, *You Are Not Your Illness*, pp. 113, adapted.

12. Gerald Sittser, *When God Doesn't Answer Your Prayers* (Grand Rapids, MI: Zondervan, 2003), pp. 53-55, adapted.

Chapter 8: Depression

1. Jon Kobat-Zinn, *The Mindful Way Through Depression* (New York: Guilford Press, 2007), p. 1.

2. Richard F. Berg, C.S.C. and Christine McCartney, *Depression and the Integrated Life* (New York: Alba House, 1981), pp. 34-35, adapted.

3. H. Norman Wright, *Winning over Your Emotions* (Eugene, OR: Harvest House, 1998), pp. 139-42, adapted.

4. Dan Blazer, "The Depression Epidemic," *Christianity Today*, March 2009, p. 29.

5. Archibald Hart, Ph.D., and Catherine Hart Ween, Ph.D., *Understanding Depression in Women* (Grand Rapids, MI: Revell, 2002), p. 41, adapted.

6. J. Raymond DePaulo, Jr., M.D., *Understanding Depression* (New York: Wiley, 2002), p. 100.

7. Ellen McGraw, *When Feeling Bad Is Good* (New York: Henry Holt & Co, 1992), pp. 34-39, adapted.

8. Ibid., p. 46.

9. Jonathan Forester, *Conquering Chronic Fatigue* (Ventura, CA: Regal Books, 2005), pp. 162-63.

10. Hart and Hart Ween, *Understanding Depression,* pp. 30-31.

11. Jane Pauley, "Depression: Out of the Shadows," *Take One Step,* TV Special, PBS, 2008.

12. Ibid., chapter 2, with Ken Duckworth, Dennis Charney, Annelle Prima, 2008.

13. Paul Meier, M.D., *Blue Genes* (Wheaton, IL: Tyndale House, 2005), pp. 37-46, adapted.

14. Ibid., p. 45.

15. Ibid., p. 26, adapted.

16. Ibid., p. 37, adapted.

17. Kobat-Zinn, *Mindful Way,* pp. 19-21, adapted.

18. Mark A. Sutton and Bruce Hennigan, M.D., *Conquering Depression* (Nashville: Broadman & Holman, 2001), pp. 91-93, adapted.

19. Ibid., p. 46.

20. DePaulo, Jr., *Understanding Depression,* pp. 177-78, adapted.

21. Pauley, "Depression: Out of the Shadows."

22. Meier, *Blue Genes,* p. 23.

23. JoAnn LeMaistre, Ph.D., *After the Diagnosis* (Dillon, CO: Alpine Guild, 1999), pp. 185-86, adapted.

24. Nancy Guthrie, *Holding On to Hope* (Wheaton, IL: Tyndale House, 2002), pp. 11-12.

25. Linda Noble Topf and Hal Zina Bennett, *You Are Not Your Illness* (New York: Simon & Schuster, 1995), p. 62.

26. Marva Dawn, *Being Well When We're Ill* (Minneapolis: Augsburg Fortress, 2008), pp. 215-16.

Chapter 9: Suffering and Pain

1. Joni Eareckson Tada and Steve Estes, *When God Weeps* (Grand Rapids, MI: Zondervan, 2000), p. 125.

2. Dwight Carlson, *When Life Isn't Fair* (Eugene, OR: Harvest House Publishers, 1989), p. 38.

3. Ibid., p. 43.

4. Delores Kuenning, *Helping People Through Grief* (Minneapolis: Bethany House, 1987), p. 203, quoting Daniel Simundson, *Where Is God in My Suffering?* (Minneapolis: Augsburg Fortress, 1983), pp. 28-29.

5. Carlson, *When Life Isn't Fair,* p. 52.

6. Harold Kushner, *When Bad Things Happen to Good People* (New York: Avon Books, 1981), p. 129.

7. Don Baker, *Pain's Hidden Purpose* (Portland, OR: Multnomah Press, 1984), p. 72.

8. Michael Card, *A Sacred Sorrow* (Colorado Springs: NavPress, 2005), p. 129.

9. Greg Barnes, *When God Interrupts* (Downer's Grove, IL: InterVarsity Press, 1996), p. 135.

10. Gerald Sittser, *When God Doesn't Answer Your Prayers* (Grand Rapids, MI: Zondervan, 2003), p. 82.

11. William Fintel and Gerald McDermott, *Cancer: A Medical and Spiritual Guide for Patients and Their Families* (Grand Rapids, MI: Baker Book House, 2004) pp. 265-75, adapted.

12. Quoted in Philip Yancey, *Where Is God When It Hurts?* (Grand Rapids, MI: Zondervan, 2002), p. 181.

13. Joshua D. Straub, "Why God? Answering Life's Most Difficult Question," *Christian Counseling Today*, 2007, vol. 15, no. 3.

14. Sittser, *When God Doesn't Answer,* pp. 127-28.

15. Larry Richards, *When It Hurts Too Much to Wait* (Dallas: Word, Inc., 1985), pp. 67-68.

16. Charles Stanley, *How to Handle Adversity* (Nashville: Thomas Nelson, 1989), p. 7.

17. Ibid., pp. 81-82.

18. Ibid., p. 171.

19. Dan B. Allender, Ph.D., and Tremper Longman, III, Ph.D., *The Cry of the Soul* (Colorado Springs: NavPress, 1994), pp. 224-34, adapted.

20. David Seamands, *Healing Grace* (Colorado Springs: Victor Books, 1988), p. 115.

Chapter 10: Rebuilding Your Life, PART 1

1. Tim Hansel, *You Gotta Keep Dancin'* (Elgin, IL: David C. Cook, 1985), pp. 47-48, 133.

2. Tommy Walker, *He Knows My Name* (Ventura, CA: Regal Books, 2004), Contents page, adapted.

3. Alexander White, as quoted by Hannah Hurnard, *Winged Life* (Wheaton, IL: Tyndale House Publishers, 1975), n.p.

4. David Burns, *Feeling Good: The New Mood Therapy* (New York: Avon Books, 1980), pp. 42-43, adapted.

5. Charlie Johnson and Denise Webster, *Recrafting a Life* (Rutledge, NY: Bruner, 2002), p. 153, adapted.

6. Ibid., p. 127.

7. Ibid., pp. 127-29, adapted.

Chapter 11: Rebuilding Your Life, PART 2

1. Don Goldenberg, M.D., *Chronic Illness and Uncertainty* (Newton Lower Falls, MA: Dorset Press, 1996), pp. 151-60, adapted.

2. Kathy Charmaz, *Good Days, Bad Days* (Brusack, NJ: Rutgers University Press, 1997), pp. 11-27, adapted.

3. Carol Sveilich, M.A., *Just Fine* (Austin: Avid Reader Press, 2005), pp. 143-47, adapted.
4. Charmaz, *Good Days, Bad Days,* p. 101.
5. Sveilich, *Just Fine,* p. 144.
6. Elizabeth Kubler-Ross, *On Death and Dying* (New York: MacMillan, 1970), n.p.
7. Charmaz, *Good Days, Bad Days,* pp. 46, 64-67, adapted.
8. John Ortberg, *When the Game Is Over, It All Goes Back in the Box* (Grand Rapids, MI: Zondervan, 2007), p. 79.
9. Craig Barnes, *When God Interrupts* (Downer's Grove, IL: InterVarsity Press, 1996), pp. 88-89.
10. Bernie Siegel, M.D., quoted in Carol Turkington, Candyce Norvell, Kim Campbell Thorton, *Hope, Faith and Healing* (Lincolnwood, IL: Publications International, 1997), pp. 61-62.
11. Ibid., pp. 91-96, adapted.

Chapter 12: Helping Others Help You

1. JoAnn LeMaistre, Ph.D., *After the Diagnosis* (Berkeley: Ulysses Press, 1995), pp. 153-56, adapted.
2. James E. Miller, *When You're the Caregiver* (Ft. Wayne, IN: Willowgreen Publishers, 1995), pp. 20-21, adapted.
3. Nina Herrmann Donnelley, *I Never Know What to Say* (New York: Ballantine Books, 1987), pp. 17-24, adapted.
4. Harold Ivan Smith, *When You Don't Know What to Say* (Kansas City, MO: Beacon Hill Press, 2002), p. 7.
5. "And the Father Will Dance," lyrics adapted from Zephaniah 3:14,17 and Psalm 54:2,4, arranged by Mark Hayes, adapted.
6. Dr. Gordon MacDonald, trauma conference, New York, 2001.

Alternative Treatments for Pain Management

1. Adapted from Loowla Khazzoom, "Alternative Treatments for Pain," copyright © 2009, published in *AARP Magazine,* Jan./Feb. 2009. Used by permission of author. All rights reserved.
2. www.mayoclinic.com/health/acupuncture/SA86, August 14, 2009.

A Pain Diary

1. James N. Dillard, M.D., D.C., with Leigh Ann Hirschman, *The Chronic Pain Solution* (New York: Bantam Books, 2002), p. 57, adapted.

Dietary Supplement Definitions

1. Paul Meier, M.D., *Blue Genes* (Wheaton, IL: Tyndale House, 2005), pp. 175-76, adapted.

More Great Books by
H. Norman Wright

101 Questions to Ask Before You Get Engaged

After You Say "I Do"

After You Say "I Do" Devotional

Before You Say "I Do"

Before You Say "I Do" Devotional

Before You Remarry

Finding the Life You've Been Looking For

Finding the Right One for You

Helping Your Kids Deal with Anger, Fear, and Sadness

Quiet Times for Couples

Quiet Times for Parents

Quiet Times for Those Who Need Comfort

Reflections of a Grieving Spouse

Gift Books

A Friend Like No Other (Dog)

My Dog Changed My Life

My Faithful Companion (Dog)

Nine Lives to Love (Cat)